◆ ◆ ◆ ◆ ◆ ◆ ◆

Kidney Health Gourmet

Diet Guide and Kidney Friendly
Recipes for People not on Dialysis

A Collection of Recipes by
Nina Kolbe RD, CSR, LD
ninakolbe@aol.com

◆ ◆ ◆ ◆ ◆ ◆ ◆ ◆

First published in 2008
Revised and updated 2010
Revised and updated 2013

Other books by this author

10 Step Diet & Lifestyle Guide for Healthier Kidneys, Avoid Dialysis

order form in back of this book

Table of Content

◆ ◆ ◆ ◆ ◆ ◆ ◆ ◆ ◆

Welcome to the Kidney Health Gourmet Diet Guide and Kidney Friendly Recipes for People not on Dialysis

Thank you for buying my cookbook. I feel as if we have embarked on a partnership that will help you manage your kidney disease while eating wonderfully delicious meals. You no longer have to worry about eating the wrong foods, as all the recipes in this book have been hand selected and analyzed to make sure they are "kidney friendly."

You may be wondering if you are alone in this diagnosis – far from it. More than 26 million Americans, 1 in 9 adults, have been diagnosed with Chronic Kidney Disease (CKD). I have worked in this field for over 20 years and I am convinced, and supported by research, that an early diagnosis, proper medical management, diet and a healthy lifestyle can all contribute to delaying the progression of kidney disease. Diabetes and high blood pressure are the most common reasons for a decrease in kidney function. I will help guide you to better manage these conditions, because this management is essential in improving the disease process.

The recipes in this book have all been carefully selected and adapted specifically for people diagnosed with Chronic Kidney Disease, but who are not on dialysis.

Consult with your doctor to better understand your kidney disease and more specific dietary needs.

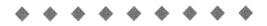

Diet and Chronic Kidney Disease

After a diagnosis of Chronic Kidney Disease, some dietary changes must be made. Specific dietary guidance to help you with the changes will be discussed in greater detail in the next few pages.

Calories

If you are a Diabetic and above your suggested body weight, slow and steady weight loss is recommended to help control your blood glucose levels. If you have *high blood pressure* and are above your suggested weight, slow and steady weight loss is also recommended. Selecting from the lower calorie recipes and increasing your activity levels will help you achieve these goals. Thirty minutes of daily exercise is recommended and has been shown to help improve *blood sugar levels* and *blood pressure.*

If you are at an appropriate weight and have found that you are eating less and experiencing unplanned weight loss, then select from the high calorie recipes. Since there are many restrictions in this diet you can add calories with foods like sugar, candy, honey, olive oil, butter, and heavy cream. If you are Diabetic, you should still limit sugar in both food and beverages made with added sugar. Your calories should come from healthy foods that give us vitamins, minerals and other important nutrients. Processed meals and snack foods should be avoided since they only contribute sodium, refined sugars, unhealthy fat and minerals that are bad for people with Diabetes, hypertension, and CKD.

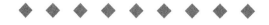

Protein

The highest sources of protein are animal products such as red meat, pork, poultry, seafood, and dairy. Smaller levels of protein are found in grains, dried beans, and vegetables. Protein is not usually limited until later stages of CKD. However, a *healthy* level of protein is recommended. A healthy level means a level more in keeping with our own physiological needs rather than restaurant supersizing. For example, a healthy 140-pound woman should consume approximately 50 grams of protein per day. This could be supplied by eating a sandwich with 2 ounces of turkey meat for lunch and a 3-ounce filet of sole for dinner. Grains, dairy, and vegetables would then supply the balance of her protein needs. For reference, 3 ounces of an animal protein looks like a deck of cards. I include many pasta dishes, rice, and casseroles that lend themselves to providing this protein serving without making the rest of your plate look empty. I also purposefully omit recipes using red meat. Research on dietary restriction of protein from red meat has found very positive results in delaying the progression of CKD in Diabetic patients. Consuming read meat has shown an increase in Albuminuria (excess protein found in the urine) in Diabetic subjects. Studies on non-Diabetic subjects have not been conclusive, but limiting red meat will not be harmful and may be very beneficial. If you cannot live without the occasional steak or hamburger try to have a modest portion size and only indulge yourself on special occasions.

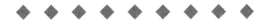

Sodium

Sodium Chloride, also known as table salt, is plentiful in our culture. Even if we do not add any sodium when cooking, it is found in huge proportions in all processed foods. Sometimes my patients ask me how they can tell if a food has been processed. I respond by asking them to tell me the natural form of a food, whether it is animal or vegetable. For example, can you picture how a cabbage grows? Yes, in the ground! Where does sauerkraut grow? If you cannot picture it then it must be processed. How about the sliced turkey in a turkey sandwich? Yes, we have all seen turkeys walking around or at least pictures of them on Thanksgiving. How about salami? Even at the Zoo I have never seen a salami animal. Get the picture? This logic can be extended to canned soups, chips, etc. If we all ate natural foods then our intake of salt would be drastically reduced. When purchasing vegetables I suggest buying fresh or frozen vegetables as opposed to canned vegetables, because the canning process adds a lot of salt. I also suggest using a wide variety of herbs and spices to flavor your meals instead of relying on salt. If you can, use fresh herbs instead of dry ones, as the taste is usually superior. There are many wonderful spice combinations at the grocery store. Read labels carefully to make sure that salt or sodium has not been added. Do not use salt substitute such as lite salt, because potassium chloride is added, which is also not recommended. You may find in these recipes that I use a lot of garlic in my cooking. Not only is the flavor wonderful, but also studies have shown that it has many health benefits. It has been shown to be effective is slowing the development of atherosclerosis and in clinical studies has shown to lower blood pressure.

Why should we worry about excess salt in our diet? Sodium has been found to increase blood pressure, which causes strains on the kidneys. Doctors suggest keeping blood pressure to the normal level of 120/80 in order to prevent the progression of CKD.

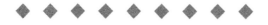

Potassium

Potassium is a mineral that regulates your heart beat and helps your muscles function well. A moderate potassium diet is recommended for early and middle stages of CKD. A lower potassium diet is recommended for later stages of CKD. A low potassium diet is approximately 2400 mg per day. The recipes in this book provide less than 500 mg of potassium each, allowing for snacks of fruits and vegetables from the lists provided. Your doctor or renal dietitian can give you more specific guidance. Remember not to use salt substitutes due to their high potassium content. I do use some higher potassium vegetables in my recipes. However, I used them in smaller quantities, and usually as part of a larger meal.

Low Potassium Vegetables: Less than 200 mg potassium per ½ cup serving	Higher Potassium Vegetables: More than 200 mg potassium per ½ cup serving
Asparagus	Artichoke
Bamboo Shoots	Black-Eyed peas
Beets	Broccoli
Cabbage	Chick peas
Carrots	Greens (collard, dandelion)
Cauliflower	Kale
Celery (1 stalk)	Kidney Beans
Corn, cooked, frozen	Parsnips
Cucumber	Peanuts
Eggplant	Potatoes
French Beans	Pumpkin
Green Onion	Rhubarb
Leek	Soybeans, fermented, green
Lettuce	Spinach
Mushrooms	Sweet potatoes

Low Potassium Vegetables: Less than 200 mg potassium per ½ cup serving	Higher Potassium Vegetables: More than 200 mg potassium per ½ cup serving
Okra	Swiss Chard
Peas	Tomatoes
Radish	
Apple 1	Apricots 2
Apple Sauce	Avocado
Blackberries	Banana
Blueberries	Cantaloupe
Cherries	Coconut raw, shredded
Cranberries	Currants
Fruit Cocktail	Dates 4
Grapefruit	Figs 2
Grapes	Guava 1
Lemon 1	Honeydew
Lime 1	Kiwi 1
Mandarin Oranges	Mango
Papaya	Nectarine 1
Peaches, canned	Orange
Pear, canned	Papaya
Pineapple	Peach, fresh
Plums 3	Persimmon 1
Pomegranate	Prunes 4
Raspberries	Raisins 3 T
Strawberries	Watermelon
Tangelo	Juices 1 cup servings: Grapefruit, Mango, Orange, Papaya, Prune

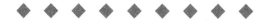

Phosphorus

Phosphorus is a mineral found in many foods, processed foods, and cola drinks. As kidney function declines removal of phosphorus from the blood may decrease. In early stages of CKD, phosphorus restriction may not be indicated. However, your doctor may suggest it in later stages. A lower phosphorus diet provides 1200-1500 mg of phosphorus per day. The recipes in this book have all been selected and modified to provide moderate to low ranges of phosphorus in each serving.

The food industry adds phosphorus to many foods to enhance flavor and add to shelf stability. Fast food restaurants also add phosphorus to chicken products. You may find "enhanced" chicken at your grocery stores. Pay attention that you are buying just a plain chicken. There are also phosphorus additives in cola drinks and some commercial iced teas. Please read labels and if you see any form of the word *phosphorus* try another brand. Recently, a patient found added phosphorus in a popular lemonade mix. Take your reading glasses to the grocery store and read the list of ingredients before making your final purchase. In my companion book Ten Step Diet & Lifestyle Guide I devote an entire chapter to phosphorus.

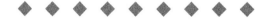

Diabetes

The goals of Diabetes management start with modest weight loss (if you are above your suggested body weight). Even a small weight loss can help improve blood glucose levels. A diet rich in fruits, vegetables, whole grains, and "good" fats is also recommended. Vigilant blood sugar management calls for up to four blood sugar checks per day. If you cannot follow that even short term at least check twice per day and rotate the times you check. Many people check only when they wake up but then they have no idea what their levels are before lunch, before dinner, etc. Rotate checking so you get an idea of your highs and lows throughout the day. Check two hours after a meal: the goal should be 140-180. Everyone should also be aware of what their glycated hemoglobin (HgA1C) is, with the goal being less than 7.5 Avoiding refined sugars from beverages, baked goods, and candy is also recommended to help stabilize blood glucose levels. This cookbook has fruits, vegetables, and natural grains as well as healthy fats. All this will contribute to better blood glucose control. Diabetes with high blood pressure put a great strain on the kidneys so both conditions should be managed vigilantly.

At the time of revision in 2013 a lower glycemic pasta is now on the market. Dreamfields Pasta. I have sampled it and found it to be delicious and I have seen much improved glucose reading from my patients when they switch to this pasta. Use this brand when making pasta dishes.

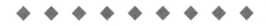

Antioxidants

Clinical studies of CKD patients show that including antioxidants in ones diet delays the progression of the disease. Cooking with olive oil and drinking tea were found to have positive effects in clinical studies. The recipes in this book use olive oil when possible and include man fruits and vegetables. Fruits and vegetables provide many different phytochemicals (plant based compounds that have been shown to reduce certain types of cancers, prevent heart disease, diabetes and reduce high blood pressure) phytochemicals act by protecting blood vessels and studies have shown that olive oil may bolster each of these benefits. Olive oil's health benefits come from the numerous plant compounds it contains. These compounds have antioxidant and anti-inflammatory effects that promote heart health, protect against cancer, and have a beneficial effect on CKD.

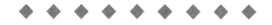

Supplementation

Over the counter use of pain relievers and anti-inflammatory medications should always be checked with your physician. The class of medicines known as non-steroidal anti-inflammatory (NSAID) is not recommended for people diagnosed with CKD. These medications are known by the following names: Ibuprofen with over the counter brands of Advil and Motrin, and the pain reliever Naproxen with the over the counter name of Aleve. Aspirin and Tylenol are generally considered safer with CKD, but again check with your doctor since Aspirin can increase your clotting time and alcohol consumption should be avoided with Tylenol use.

Vitamin and mineral use should also be carefully monitored. Over the counter multivitamin supplements may not always be appropriate with CKD. High doses of Vitamin C are not recommended due to an increase in oxalate and the formation of calcium oxalate stones. Large doses of Vitamin A are also not recommended. Supplements with potassium and phosphorus should be avoided. Many physicians are checking serum levels of Vitamin D and are prescribing supplements as necessary. Vitamin D is important for many functions in the body so make sure you find out your Vitamin D level.

The B vitamins are B1, B2, B6 B12, biotin, pantothenic acid, niacin, and Folic acid. Vitamins B1, B2, B12, niacin, pantothenic acid, and biotin should be taken in recommended daily amounts akin to the general population. Folic acid and vitamins B6 and B12 are very important vitamins that act together to promote red blood cell development. *Also, they appear to control a compound known as homocysteine, which has been identified as a possible risk factor for heart disease and stroke.* CKD patients have increased requirements for folic acid and vitamin B6, needing at least 800 mg to 1 g 600-800 mcg of folic acid and 10 mg or more of B6 each day. There are renal multivitamin preparations that your doctor can prescribe for you that will help you meet your requirements.

Most herbal medicine use has not been studied with patients diagnosed with CKD so always check with your physician regarding its use. We do know that St. John's Wort and Ginko can increase the metabolizing of other medications you may be taking.

Alfalfa, dandelion, and noni juice are all very high in potassium and should be avoided.

Chinese herbal products with aristolochic acid may be damaging to your kidneys, so its use should also be avoided. When in doubt check with your doctor.

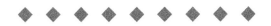

Pep Talk

There is extensive research that shows that good blood glucose control, good blood pressure control, and protein, phosphorus, and potassium modifications can help you slow down the progression of kidney disease and protect you from malnutrition. I hope you find the recipes in this book enjoyable and a tasty substitute for your favorite foods. All the recipes were tested by family and friends, and were found to be delicious for all members of the family. See your doctor regularly and your efforts at diet and exercise will help to keep you feeling great, energetic and enjoying life.

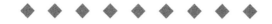

Sample Menu
For 150 lb. Female

Breakfast

1 c. cornflakes cereal

4 oz. skim milk

¾ c. fresh blueberries

coffee or tea with non-dairy creamer

Lunch

Turkey Sandwich:

2 oz. turkey

2 slices bread

1 T mayonnaise

lettuce

1 slice tomato

fresh green salad: 2 cup portion

iceberg lettuce, shredded carrots red cabbage cucumbers, onions

2 T. olive oil vinaigrette

¾ c. fresh grapes

iced tea

Snack

1 c. assorted fresh vegetables:

cucumber, celery, snow peas, radish with Chipotle Dipping Sauce

Dinner

3 oz. Honey Dijon Salmon

1 c. green beans with garlic and basil

1 c brown rice drizzled with olive oil

*1 slice Spiced Angel food cake with fresh pineapple

3 oz. red wine or water

Snack

*Jell-O with non-dairy whipped cream

*For diabetic restrictions omit Angel food cake, have fresh pineapple and sugar free Jell-O as a snack, all beverages should also be sugar free.

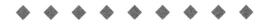

◆ ◆ ◆ ◆ ◆ ◆ ◆ ◆ ◆

Sample Menu
For 190 lb. Male

Breakfast

1 c. Rice Krispies cereal

4 oz. skim milk

1 egg

¾ c. fresh strawberries

coffee or tea with non-dairy creamer

Lunch

Roast chicken pesto sandwich:

2 oz. roast chicken

1-2 T store bought pesto or you can use mayonnaise

2 slices bread

lettuce

1 slice tomato

fresh green salad: 2 cups

iceberg lettuce, shredded carrots , red cabbage , cucumbers , onions

1-2 T olive oil vinaigrette

1 c. Greek lemon chicken and rice soup

¾ c. applesauce

iced tea or water

Snack

¾ c. assorted vegetables

2 cups raw vegetables cauliflower , cucumber , celery

¼ c dill dip

water

Dinner

3 oz. Honey Dijon Salmon

¾ c. couscous

1 c. herbed vegetables

*1 slice pound cake with ¾ c. fresh raspberries

3 oz. red wine or water

Snack

Unsalted popcorn

*For Diabetic restrictions omit pound cake and
have fresh raspberries with Cool Whip.

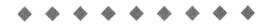

Appetizers & Beverages

Iced Tea Comparison

Acceptable Prepared Iced Teas on CKD Diet

Lipton Natural Tea

Lipton Pureleaf Tea

Turkey Hill Green Tea

Turkey Hill Raspberry Tea

Snapple Iced Teas

Arizona Green Tea

Homemade Iced Tea

Due to food additives, some teas are not recommended on the CKD diet. If you need to lose weight or are Diabetic you should opt for diet iced tea.

Not Recommended Iced Teas on CKD Diet

Lipton Brisk Iced Tea

Snapple Green Tea Citrus Fusion

Lipton Iced Tea

Lipton Green Tea Sparkling

Nestea Iced Teas

Turkey Hill Unsweetened Iced Tea

Beverage Comparison

Acceptable Beverages on CKD Diet

Water

Tea

Coffee

Clear Sodas*

Fruit Flavored Sodas*

Root Beer*

Cranberry Juice*

Apple Juice*

Grape Juice*

Country Time Lemonade*

Dasani Flavored Water*

Capri Sun*

An Italian study showed that drinking only tea, coffee, water, and 4 oz. of red wine a day slowed the progression of kidney disease. Therefore, that is what I recommend to you. The sodas and juices listed above are not harmful, but also are not beneficial to a CKD patient.

*Select diet or light if you need to lose weight or are Diabetic.

Beverages Not Recommended on the CKD Diet

Coke

Pepsi

Mr. Pibb

Hawaiian Punch Ruby Red

Orange Juice

V-8

Tropicana Fruit Drinks

Mountain Dew Code Red

Gatorade G2

Propel

Gatorade Focus

Gatorade

Amp Energy Drink

PowerAde Mountain Blast

Tang

Aquafina Flavor Splash

Vitamin Water

Sobe

Glaceau

Certain Iced Tea – see previous section

Milk Comparison

4   oz cow milk: potassium 191 mg, phosphorus 123 mg

4   oz rice milk: potassium 33 mg, phosphorus 67 mg

4   oz soy milk: potassium 143 mg, phosphorus 63 mg

4   oz unsweetened almond milk: potassium 80 mg, phosphorus   20 mg

Most people select an alternative to cow's milk if their phosphorus is elevated. If your doctor has indicated that your potassium may be elevated as well, then you may want to select the rice milk or almond milk. Please check the labels one brand of rice milk has added potassium and phosphate food additives so check labels carefully. Most CKD diets allow 4 oz of cow milk or yogurt per day. If you want to go above that then rice milk (additive free) or almond milk may be a good alternative. Soy milk is lower in phosphorus than cow milk so that may be an option if you need to lower your phosphorus intake but not potassium. There have also been some studies showing the benefit of soy in the renal diet.

Andalucia Sangria

1   bottle red wine

1   liter Sprite or Ginger Ale (diet if indicated)

1   apple peeled and chopped

Combine all ingredients in a large pitcher and chill for at least 1 hour. You can add other fruit such as berries or peaches as a garnish. Makes 16 6 oz servings.

Notes: Per serving: Calories 65, Carbohydrates 7 g, Fat 0, Protein 0, Sodium 7 mg, Potassium 73 mg, Phosphorus 8 mg.

Bellini Sangria

1   bottle white wine

½   c chopped peaches fresh or canned

1   liter Sprite or Ginger Ale (sugar free if indicated)

Combine all ingredients and chill for at least 1 hour. Makes 16 6 oz servings.

Notes: Per serving: Calories 70, Carbohydrates 7 g, Protein 0, Fat 0, Sodium 8 mg, Potassium 71 mg, Phosphorus 10 mg.

Snack Comparison

Rice Cakes made with brown rice

Popcorn Cakes

Microwave Popcorn

Tortilla Chips low fat baked

Tortilla Chips white corn

Bagel Chips

2 rice cakes: 53 mg potassium, 67 mg phosphorus, and 45 mg sodium.

2 popcorn cakes: 65 mg potassium, 55 mg phosphorus, and 58 mg sodium.

Microwave Popcorn, low fat, and low sodium, 2 cups: 68 mg potassium 75 mg phosphorus, and 139 mg sodium.

10 light, baked tortilla chips: 44 mg potassium, 51 mg phosphorus, and 160 mg sodium.

10 white corn tortilla chips, fried (the usual ones you find in large bags): 42 mg potassium, 49 mg phosphorus, and 120 mg sodium.

10 bagel chips: 37 mg potassium, 55 mg phosphorus, and 80 mg sodium.

Notes: Some of my patients have been buying the "healthy" vegetable or Terra Chips. These are extremely high in potassium content! Always check your chips for food additives, which are very unhealthy for your kidneys.

Cheese Comparison

Hard cheeses per 1 oz
American: 94 calories, 6 g protein, 7 g fat, 274 mg sodium, 103 mg potassium, 11 mg phosphorus

Cheddar: 114 calories, 7 g protein, 9 g fat, 175 mg sodium, 28 mg potassium, 145 mg phosphorus

Monteray Jack: 104 calories, 7 g protein, 8 g fat, 150 mg sodium, 23 mg potassium, 124 mg phosphorus

Note: American cheese and Cottage cheese contain phosphorus food

Soft cheeses per 1 oz
Brie: 95 calories, 6 g protein, 8 g fat, 172 mg sodium, 43 mg potassium, 53 mg phosphorus

Cream Cheese: 96 calories, 2 g protein, 9 g fat, 91 mg sodium, 39 mg potassium, 30 mg phosphorus

Feta: 75 calories, 4 g protein, 6 g fat, 316 mg sodium, 18 mg potassium, 95 mg phosphorus

2% Cottage Cheese: 97 calories, 13 g protein, 3 g fat, 373 mg sodium, 95 mg potassium, 184 mg phosphorus

Add cheese to your diet as a dessert or a garnish for the main meal — eat it in moderation.

Notes: American cheese and Cottage cheese contain phosphorus food additives. This means the phosphorus in those cheeses is more readily absorbed into the blood stream than the phosphorus that occurs naturally in other types of cheese. Therefore, you should consume American and Cottage cheese less than other types of cheese.

Turkey Roll Up

4	10 inch flour tortillas
8	slices deli turkey
1	T mayonnaise low fat
2	oz low fat cream cheese at room temperature
2	T cranberry sauce
	lettuce

Place tortillas in a paper towel and microwave for 30-45 seconds until the tortillas are warm and soft. Meanwhile, mix softened cream cheese, mayonnaise, and cranberry sauce in a bowl until well blended. Place the 4 tortillas on a work surface. Spread ¼ of the cream cheese mixture onto each tortilla. Cover this with 2 slices of deli turkey and a large lettuce leaf. Roll up the tortillas like a taco and refrigerate until set.

If serving as appetizers, cut each tortilla in half and place on a plate seam side down.

Notes: Per tortilla: Calories 340, Carbohydrates 56 g, Protein 11 g, Fat 7 g, Sodium 250 mg, Potassium 208 mg, Phosphorus 170 mg.

Fiesta Roll-Ups

4	oz can green chilies, chopped
2	garlic cloves, crushed
½	tsp ground cumin
½	tsp chili powder (or more to taste)
4	T green onions, thinly sliced
8	oz pkg cream cheese, softened (use light for lower calories)
6	8" flour tortillas

Combine green chilies, garlic, cumin, chili powder, and onions in a bowl. Blend in softened cream cheese. Spread a thin layer of cream cheese mixture onto each tortilla leaving a ¼ inch edge uncovered. Roll up like a jellyroll. Use a toothpick to secure the rolls. Cover and refrigerate for at least 1 hour. Slice rolls into 1" pieces and serve as a snack or appetizer.

Notes: 4 pieces 1" each: Calories 126, Carbohydrates 12 g, protein 3 g, Fat 7 g, Sodium 47 mg, Potassium 47 mg, Phosphorus 26 mg.

Quick Salmon Spread

A fatty fish such as salmon should be part of your meal plan at least twice per week. The whole family will benefit from the Omega Fatty Acids.

1	15 oz can red salmon, drained
¼	c celery, finely chopped
¼	c onion, finely chopped
2	T low fat mayonnaise
1	tsp lemon juice
½	tsp dried dill
¼	tsp paprika
⅛	tsp Worcestershire sauce

Combine all ingredients in a blender or food processor. Cover and blend until smooth. Transfer to a bowl and chill for at least 1 hour. Serve on unsalted crackers or Melba round toasts. Makes 2 cups.

Notes: Per 1 T (Spread only): Calories 21, Carbohydrates 1 g, Protein 2 g, Fat 1 g, Sodium 60 mg, Potassium 48 mg, Phosphorus 39 mg.

Smoked Salmon Canape

¾ c light cream cheese, softened

½ c red onion, chopped

1 T fresh dill and loose sprigs for garnish

2 tsp prepared horseradish

   Black pepper to taste

½ lb thinly sliced smoked salmon

   small, thin pumpernickel bread pieces

In a small bowl combine cream cheese, onion, chopped dill, and horseradish. Stir well and season with pepper. Cover the bread pieces with a layer of the cream cheese mixture; lay a piece of salmon over that and top with a sprig of dill. Makes enough for 24 canapés.

Notes: Per canapé: Calories 27, Carbohydrates 4 g, Protein 2 g, Fat 2 g, Sodium 89 mg, Potassium 33 mg, Phosphorus 45 mg.

Puffy Shrimp Toast

5	oz shrimp, peeled and deveined
2	T green onions, chopped
1	T teriyaki sauce
1	T dry sherry
1½	tsp peanut oil
¼	tsp sesame oil
¼	tsp fresh ginger, minced
1	egg white
2	slices white bread cut in half to make 8 triangles

Place raw shrimp on a cutting board and finely chop. Transfer to a bowl. Add scallions, teriyaki sauce, sherry, peanut oil, sesame oil, and ginger. Mix well. Preheat oven to 350º F. In a glass bowl beat egg white until it is stiff but not dry. Spread 1/8 of the shrimp mixture and 1/8 of the beaten egg white onto each triangle toast. Make sure to cover all of the shrimp mixture. Arrange bread triangles on a non-stick baking sheet and bake until shrimp mixture is cooked through and topping is lightly browned, about 10-15 minutes. Serves 4, 2 triangles each.

Notes: Per serving: Calories 67, Carbohydrates 7 g, Protein 4 g, Fat 3 g, Sodium 250 mg, Potassium 53 mg, Phosphorus 42 mg.

Greek Layer Dip

10   oz tub of commercially prepared hummus such as
Sabra or Sheik brand

2   large cucumbers, peeled and diced

1½ T olive oil

1   T lemon juice

    oregano and pepper to taste

2   T chopped tomato

2   T chopped feta cheese

Peel cucumbers and chop, blotting out excess moisture with a paper towel. In a bowl mix olive oil, lemon juice, oregano, and pepper to create the dressing. Whisk to combine. Add dressing to cucumbers and toss. On a large flat plate arrange the hummus in a thin layer, and top with a layer of cucumbers. Garnish with 2 T of chopped tomatoes and 2 T of feta cheese. Serve with cut up pita wedges. A serving is 4-inch whole-wheat pita cut into slices and 4 T of hummus, cucumber dip.

Some bread has more phosphorus than others. For example, whole wheat bread has more phosphorus than white bread. Due to their higher fiber and better nutritional composition, I do not restrict whole wheat bread. However, if you are concerned about your phosphorus intake then unleavened breads such as pita or the Indian Naan breads are your healthiest options.

Notes: Per serving: 4 T hummus dip: Calories 40, Carbohydrates 5.1 g, Protein 2 g, Fat 2.5 g, Sodium 57 mg, Potassium 34 mg, Phosphorus 26 mg.

Per serving: 1 4" whole wheat pita wedge: Calories 74, Carbohydrates 15 g, Protein 2.7 g, Fat 2 g, Sodium 149 mg, Potassium 48 mg, Phosphorus 50 mg.

Mushrooms Stuffed With Herb Cheese

18	medium mushrooms
3	T whipped cream cheese
1	T fresh parsley, chopped
1	T fresh basil leaves, chopped
2	tsp Parmesan cheese, grated
1	garlic clove, peeled and minced
2	tsp plain breadcrumbs

Preheat over to 450º F. Wash mushrooms, remove and chop mushroom stems, reserving the caps. In a small mixing bowl use a fork to combine the chopped mushrooms, cream cheese, parsley, basil, Parmesan cheese, and garlic. Mix well. Fill each reserved mushroom cap with an equal amount of the cream cheese mixture (about 1 tsp) and arrange on a nonstick baking pan. Sprinkle breadcrumbs over each stuffed mushroom. Pour ¼ cup water in the bottom of the pan and bake until the mushrooms are fork-tender and lightly browned, about 8-10 minutes. Makes 4 servings, 4 mushrooms each.

Notes: Per serving: Calories 75, Carbohydrates 5 g, Protein 4 g, Fat 5 g, Sodium 111 mg, Potassium 213 mg, Phosphorus 89 mg.

Chipotle Dipping Sauce

¾   c sour cream (use low fat if trying to limit calories)

¼   c blue cheese, crumbled

2   tsp Mrs. Dash Southwest Chipotle Seasoning Blend

Combine all ingredients and chill until ready to serve. Serving size 1-2 T.

Notes: Per 1 T: Calories 31, Carbs 3 g, Fat 3 g, Protein 0 Sodium 8 mg, Potassium 21 mg, Phosphorus 12 mg.

Cucumber Dill Dip

1   large cucumber

2   c sour cream (use light if want to limit calories)

1   tsp dried dill or 3 T fresh dill

    pepper to taste

Peel cucumber, halve lengthwise, remove seeds and chop finely or grate. Squeeze excess liquid from grated cucumber. Mix with sour cream, pepper and dill weed. Refrigerate for 1-2 hours before serving.

You can add onions to this recipe for a bit more punch.

Notes: Per 1 T serving: Calories 31, Carbs 2 g, Fat 3 g, Sodium 8 mg, Phosphorus 12 mg, Potassium 21 mg.

Sour Cream Pesto Dip

1   c sour cream (use low fat if trying to limit calories)

½   c basil pesto – can use store bought

3   T grated Parmesan cheese

Combine all the ingredients and mix well to blend. Serve chilled with raw vegetables suggested in the sample menu or under potassium table.

Notes: Per 1 T serving: Calories 33, Fat 3 g, Carbs 2 g, Sodium 9 mg, Potassium 22 mg, Phosphorus 9 mg.

Mrs. Dash Sour Cream Yogurt Dip

1	c sour cream (use low fat if trying to limit calories)
½	c plain yogurt
¼	c mayonnaise
2	T Mrs. Dash Original Blend
½	tsp sugar

Combine all ingredients in a small bowl and mix well. Cover and chill for 1-2 hours or overnight to let flavors settle.

Mrs. Dash has a wide variety of seasoning blends, which you should look at and experiment with to bring out the flavor in food.

Notes: Per 1 T serving: Calories 45, Carbohydrates 2 g, Protein 1 g, Fat 3 g, Sodium 50 mg, Potassium 60 mg, Phosphorus 24 mg.

Soups & Salads

Commercial Soup Comparison

Commercial Condensed Chicken Mushroom Soup

Commercial Split Pea Soup

Commercial Chicken Vegetable Soup

Commercial Chicken Noodle Soup

1 **can** of chicken mushroom soup: 374 mg potassium, 65 mg phosphorus, and 2289 mg sodium (I know, I just report the facts).

1 **can** split pea soup: 463 mg potassium, 137 mg phosphorus, and 420 mg sodium.

1 **cup** chicken vegetable soup: 369 mg potassium, 109 mg phosphorus, and 89 mg sodium.

1 **cup** chicken noodle soup: 76 mg potassium, 49 mg phosphorus, and 815 mg sodium.

I am an advocate for home made soups, because you really cut back on sodium and all food additives, which are not good for your kidneys. However, in some instances canned soup may be a reality for you, so I went through different soups and found the best ones.

(continued)

Amy's Organic Soups meeting CKD criteria:

    Lentil Soup

    Vegetable Barley Soup

    Light in Sodium Minestrone Soup

    Light in Sodium Lentil Soup

Notes: You may be wondering what is more important: potassium or sodium? If your potassium is elevated then it takes priority over all other restrictions.

Vegetable Consomme

3   large carrots, coarsely chopped

1   turnip, chopped

2   celery stalks, chopped

2   onions, peeled and chopped

2   T olive oil

½   c fresh parsley

1   bay leaf

1   tsp thyme leaves

      garlic and peppercorns to taste

Scrub and chop carrots, turnip, celery, and onions. Heal olive oil in an 8 qt pot. Add chopped vegetables and cook over medium heat stirring often for 15 minutes. Add 3 quarts of water, parsley, bay leaf, and thyme leaves. Add garlic and peppercorns to taste. Cover and bring to a boil. Reduce heat and simmer for 1½ hours. Strain and discard vegetables. Recipe makes 2 ½ quarts stock.

Notes: Per serving: Calories 20, Carbohydrates 3 g, Protein 1 g, fat 0, Sodium 23 mg, Potassium 53 mg, Phosphorus 14 mg.

Homemade Chicken Broth

2   lbs chicken necks and backs for stock

1   celery stalk, cut into ½ inch lengths

2   small carrots, peeled and diced

1   yellow onion, cut in half

1   leek, washed and sliced

2   green onions, cut into 2 inch lengths

1   bay leaf

     pepper to taste

Combine chicken pieces, celery, carrots, yellow onions, leek, green onion, bay leaf, and pepper to taste in a 4-quart saucepan. Add cold water to fill the pan ¾ full. Place over medium heat, uncovered, and bring slowly to a boil. Skim off any fat that forms on the surface. Reduce heat to low and simmer, uncovered, for 2 ½ hours. Strain through a colander to keep the broth and adjust seasonings. Refrigerate and remove fat that collects on the top. Can be frozen and used in future recipes.

Add fresh ginger to this recipe to give the soup an Asian flavor.

The recipes in this book frequently call for chicken broth or Asian chicken broth. I suggest having some on hand in the freezer in small containers and thawing them as you need it.

Notes: Calories 38, Carbohydrates 6 g, Fat 1 g, Protein 3 g, Sodium 18 mg, Potassium 90 mg, Phosphorus 29 mg.

Arizona Harvest Soup

8	oz cooked black beans
7	cups home made chicken broth (page 45) or low sodium broth
8	oz canned crushed tomatoes
2	cups finely chopped onion
1	whole jalapeno
1	rib celery, finely diced
2	carrots, chopped
2	cloves garlic, peeled and minced
1	bay leaf
2	tsp ground cumin
¾	tsp ground oregano
½	tsp coriander
1	tsp black pepper
⅛	tsp ground cloves
¾	c brown rice
2	small zucchinis, diced
1½	T dried basil

Put chicken broth in a large saucepan over high heat. Add black beans, whole can of crushed tomatoes including liquid, 1 c onions, carrots, celery, jalapeno, garlic, bay leaf, cumin, oregano, coriander, and black pepper. Stir well. When this comes to a boil reduce heat and simmer for 30 minutes. In a

(continued)

separate pan, heat oil on high. Add rice, the other 1 c onions, garlic, zucchini, and basil. Cook for 5-10 minutes. Add the rice mixture to the chicken broth mixture and simmer another 30 minutes. Remove jalapeno and bay leaf. Adjust seasonings. I personally like a very bold taste to my food so I am liberal with cumin, pepper, and garlic. Makes 7 meal-sized servings. You can add ground turkey (browned first in a saucepan) to the soup to make it a main meal soup.

Occasionally, I do provide you with recipes using dried beans, which you may know are not recommended for the kidney disease diet due to their phosphorus and potassium content. In this recipe 8 oz of beans is split into 7 servings making it an acceptable meal.

Notes: Calories 138, Carbohydrates 28 g, Protein 5 g, Fat 1 g, Sodium 366 mg, Potassium 343 mg, Phosphorus 142 mg.

Chipotle Turkey And Corn Soup

1	T olive oil
1	lb ground turkey
2	tsp chilies in adobo sauce
28	oz homemade chicken broth (page 46) or commercial low sodium soup
1	14 oz cream style corn
¼	c fresh cilantro, chopped
½	c crushed lime flavored tortilla chips

Heat olive oil in a large saucepan over medium-high heat. Add ground turkey; cook for 3 minutes or until browned, stirring occasionally. Stir in adobo sauce, chilies, chicken broth, and corn. Bring to a boil. Reduce heat to medium low and simmer for 5 minutes. Stir in 3 T cilantro. Divide evenly among 4 bowls and sprinkle with remaining cilantro and chips. Serves 4; serving size 1 ½ c.

Notes: Per serving: Calories 189, Carbohydrates 25 g, Protein 11 g, Fat 5 g, Sodium 420 mg, Potassium 282 mg, Phosphorus 141 mg.

Greek Lemon Chicken Soup

8	c homemade chicken broth (page 45)
½	c uncooked white rice
4	T flour
4	T melted butter
3½	oz lemon juice
¾	c finely chopped chicken meat
1	T parsley

Combine broth and rice in 3-quart pot and simmer for 30 minutes. Combine flour and butter in separate saucepan. Cook low heat, stirring for 5 minutes. Stir butter mixture into stock, and heat until thickened. Stir in lemon juice slowly, add chicken and garnish with parsley. Makes 9 servings of ½ c.

Notes: Calories 101, Protein 6g, Fat 3.3g, Carbohydrates 14 g, Sodium 60 mg, Potassium 64 mg, and Phosphorus 39 mg.

Lettuce Potassium Comparison

Per 1 cup serving size:

ICEBERG LETTUCE: 110 mg potassium

BOSTON LETTUCE: 238 mg potassium

ROMAINE LETTUCE: 247 mg potassium

ARUGULA LETTUCE: 269 mg potassium

SPINACH LEAVES RAW: 167 mg potassium

Note: The main ingredient that you have to be mindful about when consuming lettuce is the amount of potassium it provides. You can see that if you have been told to "watch" your potassium then Iceberg lettuce is your best option. For those who say it is flavorless, perhaps mixing it with a bit of your favorite lettuce might give you additional flavor without consuming excessive potassium.

Waldorf Coleslaw

3	c shredded cabbage
3	c Granny Smith apples, peeled and diced
5	T dried cranberries
3	T fat free plain yogurt
2	T low fat mayonnaise
1	T honey
1	tsp prepared horseradish
¼	tsp black pepper

Combine cabbage, apples, and cranberries in a bowl. Combine yogurt and the remaining ingredients in another bowl, stirring well with a whisk. Pour over yogurt mixture over cabbage mixture and toss to combine. Cover and chill for 2 hours. Makes 10 servings, ½ c each.

Notes: Per ½ c serving: Calories 55, Carbohydrates 9 g, Fat 1.8 g, Protein 1 g, Sodium 60 mg, Potassium 101 mg, Phosphorus 25 mg.

Broccoli Slaw

½   c sugar

½   c white vinegar

⅓   c olive oil

¼   c hot water

2   packets Oriental Ramen Noodles

2   packages broccoli slaw mixture (sold at most supermarkets)

2   bunches scallions

Mix together the sugar, vinegar, and seasoning packets from the Ramen noodles. Add olive oil then hot water. Combine with broccoli slaw and scallions. Do not add the noodles yet. Chill for 2 hours. Just before serving add the ramen noodles so they are nice and crunchy. Makes 16 servings.

Ramen noodles are deadly in sodium, but because they are divided between 16 servings it makes them more reasonable. This is a favorite recipe of mine and I hope you try it.

Notes: Per serving: Calories 100, Carbohydrates 1 g, Fat 6 g, Protein 1 g, Sodium 270 mg, Potassium 46 mg, Phosphorus 33 m

Asian Coleslaw

3½   c shredded Napa cabbage

½   c shredded red cabbage

½   c green onions

½   c fresh cilantro

½   c frozen green peas, thawed

1½   T sesame seeds

½   c low fat mayonnaise

1½   T white wine vinegar

2   tsp low sodium soy sauce

½   tsp sesame oil

¼   tsp ground pepper

¼   c sliced almonds

Combine Napa cabbage, red cabbage, green onions, cilantro, peas, and sesame seeds in a large bowl. Combine mayonnaise, vinegar, soy sauce, sesame oil, and pepper in a separate bowl, stirring with a whisk. Add mayonnaise mixture to cabbage mixture, and toss well to combine. Sprinkle with almonds. Cover and chill for at least 1 hour before serving. Makes 6 servings about 2/3 c each.

Notes: Per serving: Calories 97, Fat 7 g, Protein 3 g, Carbohydrates 7 g, Sodium 133 mg, Potassium 219 mg, Phosphorus 68 mg.

Curried Chicken Salad

3   c chicken, cooked and diced

¼   c red onion, finely chopped

¼ - ½ c plain fat free yogurt

3   T low fat mayonnaise

1   T honey

1   c grapes, cut in half

1   T curry powder

1   tsp pepper

Combine chicken and onions in a large bowl. In a separate bowl combine yogurt, mayonnaise, honey, and curry. Add the yogurt, mayonnaise, honey, and curry to chicken mixture and mix gently. Add grapes and adjust pepper and curry to taste. Makes 6 servings.

Notes: Per serving: Calories 159, Carbohydrates 11 g, Protein 19 g, Fat 4 g, Sodium 132 mg, Potassium 261 mg, phosphorus 201 mg.

Risotto And Salmon Salad

1	c uncooked Italian Arborizo rice (risotto rice)
12	oz uncooked salmon steaks
1½	c frozen green peas, thawed
½	c cucumber, peeled and diced
¼	c scallions
3	T fresh dill, chopped
1	T fresh mint, finely chopped
1	tsp grated lemon zest
⅓	c olive oil
¼	c lemon juice
1	garlic clove, crushed
	pepper to taste
	fresh dill for garnish

Boil 2 cups of water; once boiling add rice. Cover and cook over low heat for 12-15 minutes, or until the water is absorbed and the rice is tender. Let stand uncovered until the rice has cooled. Broil the salmon steaks until cooked, about 15 minutes. When done, put the steaks on a plate and allow them to cool. To make the dressing, whisk the oil, lemon juice, garlic, pepper, and dill together in a small bowl. Spoon about 2 T of the dressing over the salmon, cover and refrigerate until ready to serve. Combine rice, peas, cucumber, scallions, dill, mint, and lemon zest in a serving bowl. Add the remaining lemon and dill dressing and toss to coat. Add the salmon (cut into 1" pieces) and gently mix in to keep the salmon from breaking apart. Garnish with sprigs of fresh dill and you are ready to serve.

(continued)

At times fresh and dried herbs can be substituted, but fresh dill really makes this recipe so do try and find it. Makes 4 servings.

Notes: Per serving: Calories 268, Carbohydrates 20 g, Fat 9 g, Protein 14 g, Sodium 79 mg, Potassium 334 mg, Phosphorus 193 mg.

Greek Style Couscous Salad

2	c water	
1½	c dried couscous	
¾	c garbanzo beans, from a can	
⅔	c red onion, chopped	
⅔	c black olives, sliced	
6	T fresh mint	
4	T olive oil	
3	T lemon juice	
6	oz feta cheese, crumbled	

Bring water to a boil, add the couscous, cover and take off the heat. The couscous will have absorbed the water in approximately 10-14 minutes. Fluff the couscous with a fork; add the garbanzo beans, olive oil, onion, olives, mint, and lemon juice. Mix well, add feta and toss again. Season with pepper, refrigerate until ready to serve. Serves 6.

Notes: Per serving: Calories 285, Carbohydrates 41 g, Protein 13 g, Fat 6 g, Sodium 319 mg, Potassium 249 mg, Phosphorus 249 mg.

Greek Orzo And Shrimp Salad

6	c water
1½	lb box orzo
1½	bunches green onions, chopped
½	lb feta cheese, crumbled
3	T fresh dill, chopped
7	T lemon juice
6	T olive oil
2	lbs uncooked medium shrimp, peeled and deveined
2	c cucumber, peeled and chopped

Bring water to a boil, add the orzo and cook for about 10 minutes. Drain and rinse with cold water. Transfer to a large bowl; add green onion, feta cheese, chopped dill, lemon juice, and olive oil. Mix well. Cook shrimp in boiling water until pink, about 2 minutes. Drain and rinse in cold water. Mix into salad, season with pepper. Cover and refrigerate. Mix cucumbers into salad before serving. Garnish with dill and feta. Makes 20 servings.

Notes: Per serving: Calories 129, Carbohydrates 9 g, Protein 5 g, Fat 8 g, Sodium 105 mg, Potassium 64 mg, Phosphorus 72 mg.

Bulgur Salad With Oriental Dressing

2	c water
¾	c bulgur wheat
1¼	c red cabbage, thinly sliced
½	c shredded carrots
1	c seedless red grapes
¼	c red peppers, chopped
½	c green onions
½	c fresh parsley, chopped
⅓	c rice vinegar
2	T peanut oil
1	T low sodium soy sauce
1	T oriental soy sauce
1	tsp Dijon prepared mustard
	cilantro as a garnish

Bring 2 cups water to a boil in a medium saucepan. Stir in bulgur, cover and remove from heat. Let stand until softened, about 15 minutes. Drain bulgur, transfer to a large bowl, add cabbage, carrots, grapes, red pepper, green onions, and parsley; toss to combine. Blend vinegar, peanut oil, soy sauce, sesame oil, and mustard in a blender. Pour over salad and toss to coat. Cover and refrigerate. Can be prepared one day ahead. Garnish with cilantro. Makes 6 servings.

Notes: Per serving: Calories 125, Carbohydrates 21 g, Protein 3 g, Fat 4 g, Sodium 87 mg, Potassium 226 mg, Phosphorus 85 mg.

Beet And Goat Cheese Salad

- 2   beets, cooked (can use canned or already roasted)
- 2   oz soft goat cheese
- 2   c lettuce (1 c iceberg and 1 c your choice)
- ¼   tsp honey
- 1   tsp prepared Dijon mustard
- ½   c lemon juice
- ½   c olive oil
- 2   T crushed pistachios

Prepare 4 salad plates. Mix lettuce and place on plates, slice beets and distribute them equally between the 4 plates. Place cheese on top of beets. Mix lemon juice, mustard, and honey in a blender. Add olive oil slowly in a steady but slow stream. Drizzle dressing over the salads and garnish with crushed pistachios.

If you like to eat a lot of lettuce then I suggest mainly eating Iceberg lettuce, because it is the lowest potassium option. See lettuce comparison section for more details.

Notes: Per serving: Calories 238, Carbohydrates 12 g, Fat 15 g, Protein 7 g, Sodium 146 mg, Potassium 261 mg, Phosphorus 103 mg.

Lentil And Bulgur Salad

1   c lentils

4¼ c homemade chicken broth (page 45) or low sodium
       store- bought broth, divided

1   c bulgur

½   red onion, finely chopped

1   c fresh parsley, minced

½   c scallions, chopped

2   garlic cloves, minced

1   T prepared Dijon mustard

1   T olive oil

2   T balsamic vinegar

½   tsp Worcestershire sauce

¼   tsp hot pepper sauce (Tabasco)

1   tsp dried oregano

1   tsp dried basil

       black pepper to taste

½   tsp ground cumin

In a medium pan cook the lentils in 4 cups of chicken broth for 30 minutes. Let the lentils stand for another 10 minutes, then drain them. Meanwhile, put the bulgur in a heatproof bowl, pour hot water over it, let stand 10 minutes and then drain it. Combine the lentils and bulgur in a large bowl, and then add onions and parsley. In a small bowl combine the dressing ingredients (garlic, mustard, ¼ c chicken broth, olive oil, balsamic vinegar, Worcestershire sauce, Tabasco sauce, oregano, basil, black pepper, and cumin.) Whisk briskly and pour over the lentil mixture; toss well. Add the scallions before serving. Makes 6 1 cup servings.

Notes: Per serving: Calories 216, Carbohydrates 38 g, Protein 11 g, Fat 3 g, Sodium 40 mg, Potassium 300 mg, Phosphorus 169 mg.

Tabbouleh With Lentils

¾   c lentils

5   c water, divided

½   c bulgur wheat

1   pinch allspice

1   c cucumber, peeled and chopped

½   c diced tomatoes (1 medium tomato)

¼   c mint leaves, chopped

¼   c parsley

½   c scallions, chopped

¼   c fresh lemon juice

¼   c olive oil

   pepper to taste

   iceberg lettuce

Parboil the lentils in 4 c of water for 40 minutes, and then drain. Wash the bulgur whet in cold water, drain, and combine with the lentils in a bowl. Bring 1 cup of water to a boil with the allspice. Add the bulgur and lentil mixture. Allow the bulgur and lentil mixture to soak until all the liquid is absorbed, about 30 minutes to 1 hour (depending on the type of bulgur). If the bulgur is tender but some water remains, drain off the excess water. Add cucumber, garlic, tomato, mint, parsley, scallions, lemon juice, and olive oil.

Toss to combine, add pepper to taste, and chill. Serve on a bed of lettuce and garnish with lemon slices.

If you have done your homework you are probably saying, "I thought tomatoes are not recommended for a CKD diet". Tomatoes are high in potassium so foods made with tomato sauce are usually too high in potassium to have made this book. But in this case you have 1 tomato split into 6 servings, so the amount of potassium is acceptable.

Notes: Per serving: Calories 270, Carbohydrates 39 g, Protein 9 g, Fat 7 g, Sodium 18 mg, Potassium 213 mg, Phosphorus 161 mg.

Cucumber Mint Salad

2   large cucumbers, peeled, seeded, and thinly sliced

1   T fresh mint leaves, minced and whole leaves for garnish

½   red onion, chopped

½   c plain low fat or fat free yogurt

1   T cider vinegar

1   tsp lemon juice

1   tsp white wine or water

      pepper to taste

In a medium bowl toss the cucumbers with the mint, set aside. In a small bowl combine the yogurt, onion, vinegar, lemon juice, wine or water, and pepper. Pour the dressing over the cucumber-mint mixture and toss to coat. Chill for at least 1 hour, garnish with mint leaves. Makes 4 servings.

Notes: Per serving: Calories 26, Carbohydrates 5 g, Fat 1 g, Protein 2 g, Sodium 24 mg, Potassium 175 mg, Phosphorus 62 mg.

Thai Cucumber Salad

⅓   c shallot, minced

⅓   c green onions, sliced

4   medium cucumbers, peeled in half, seeded, and thinly sliced

2-4 hot red chilies, seeded and thinly sliced

½   c rice vinegar

2   T sugar

¼   c fresh cilantro

Combine shallots, onions, cucumbers, and chilies in a large bowl. Combine vinegar and sugar in a small bowl, and stir well. Add the small bowl to the cucumber mixture and toss to coat. Stir in cilantro. Makes 10 servings, each ½ c.

Notes: Per serving: Calories 30, Carbohydrates 7 g, Protein 0.8 g, Fat 0 g, Sodium 5 mg, Potassium 103 mg, Phosphorus 15 mg.

Wedge Salad With Blue Cheese Dressing

This simple salad is a staple at many steakhouses, and it is one of my personal favorites.

Blue Cheese Dressing

8	oz plain low fat yogurt
¾	c buttermilk
2	oz blue cheese
1	tsp cider vinegar
¼	tsp black pepper
1	garlic clove, minced

Spoon the yogurt onto several paper towels. Spread the yogurt to ½ inch thickness. Cover with additional paper towels. Let stand 5 minutes. Scrape into a bowl, add buttermilk and remaining ingredients, stir well. Cover and chill until ready to serve.

(continued)

Salad

1	head of Iceberg lettuce, cut into 4 wedges
4	slices turkey bacon
2	oz blue cheese
1	small tomato, chopped

Tear the outside leaves that may not be crisp from the head of lettuce and discard. Cut the remaining lettuce into large wedges at least 5 inches long. Microwave turkey bacon on a paper towel for 30 seconds, take out of the microwave oven and blot extra fat. Place the salad on a plate and garnish with tomato, cheese crumbles, and 1 slice of crumbled turkey bacon.

Drizzle dressing over salad and serve. The above ingredients serve 4.

I also want to use this opportunity to give you a comparison of the different lettuces. The main mineral that you are looking to minimize is potassium. Per cup, iceberg provides 140 mg; Romaine lettuce provides 247 mg; Boston 238 mg; Arugula 368 mg; and red leaf 187 mg. If you love salads and want to eat large quantities of lettuce then I suggest using primarily Iceberg lettuce.

Notes: Per serving with 1 T dressing: Calories 115, Carbohydrates 10 g, Protein 3 g, Fat 5 g, Sodium 100 mg, Potassium 190 mg, Phosphorus 75 mg.

Tuna And White Bean Mediterranean Salad

8	oz tuna, packed in water, drained and rinsed
4	oz white kidney beans (cannellini beans), drained and rinsed
4	T celery, finely chopped
2	T red onion, finely chopped
2	T fresh parsley, minced
4	T homemade chicken broth (page 45) or store-bought low sodium chicken broth
1	T olive oil
1	T red wine vinegar
2	tsp water
	pepper to taste

In a salad bowl combine tuna, beans, celery, onions, and parsley. Toss to combine. Using a wire whisk, combine broth, oil, vinegar, water, and pepper in a small mixing bowl. Pour over tuna mixture and toss to coat. Cover and refrigerate until ready to serve. Makes 4 servings.

Tuna and salmon are two of the healthiest fish due to their huge amounts of Omega Fatty Acids. I recommend 2 servings per week of these deep-sea fatty fish.

Notes: Per serving: Calories 180, Carbohydrates 16 g, Protein 14 g, Fat 6 g, Sodium 162 mg, Potassium 305 mg, Phosphorus 205 mg.

Olive Oil Herb Dressing

1	T fresh parsley
1	c chives, cut into 1" pieces
1	clove garlic, minced
2	T Dijon style mustard
¾	c extra virgin olive oil
¼	c red wine vinegar
3	T lemon juice
2	tsp anchovy paste (optional)

Blend parsley, chives, and garlic in a blender or food processor. Add remaining ingredients and blend until smooth.

Notes: Serving size is 1-3 T depending on your preference. This recipe is a negligible source of potassium, phosphorus, and sodium. Provides approximately 100 calories per 2 T serving.

Simple Balsamic Vinaigrette

¼   c balsamic vinegar

2   tsp brown sugar or honey

1   T garlic, chopped

     black pepper to taste

1   tsp Mrs. Dash Italian seasoning

¾   c olive oil

Beat vinegar in a bowl with sugar or honey until sugar dissolves or honey combines with vinegar. Add garlic and Mrs. Dash seasoning. Add oil a little bit at a time, beating constantly or place in a screw top jar and shake to combine ingredients.

Using a superior quality balsamic vinegar really makes the vinaigrette fabulous.

Notes: This dressing has no significant sources of any mineral or nutrient besides calories and fat. Per T: Calories 72, Fat 7 g.

Vegetables & Side Dishes

Leached Mashed Potatoes

Soaking potatoes reduces the potassium content by about a third. You can also use soaked potatoes to make home fries and baked potato wedges. You can use this method for sweet potatoes or yams as well.

2	large baking potatoes, peeled and cut into large pieces
3	cloves garlic
2	T reduced fat sour cream
1	T fresh butter
2	oz milk
	pepper to taste
	salt to taste

To prepare the potatoes, peel and cut them into large chunks. Place them in a bowl and submerge them in cold water. Refrigerate the potato chunks overnight. When ready to make the mashed potatoes drain the water. Place the potatoes in a pot of water, add garlic cloves and bring to a boil. Cook until soft, about 20 minutes. Drain the water, but not the garlic and add sour cream, butter, and 2 oz hot milk to the potatoes; mix. Add pepper and a dash of salt to taste. Makes 4 1cup servings.

Notes: Per serving: Calories 105, Carbohydrates 15 g, Protein 2 g, Fat 5 g, Sodium 45 mg, Potassium 122 mg, Phosphorus 38

Garlic Green Beans

1	lb fresh green beans with ends trimmed (can use frozen)
1	c breadcrumbs
3	cloves garlic, minced
¼	tsp black pepper
2	tsp sesame seeds
3	T olive oil

Steam green beans until tender. Set aside. In a skillet, sauté garlic and sesame seeds in olive oil. Add breadcrumbs and pepper; sauté until the crumbs are brown. Toss with the green beans and serve. Makes 6 servings.

Notes: Per serving: Calories 111, Carbohydrates 19 g, Protein 2 g, Fat 7 g, Sodium 43 mg, Potassium 156 mg, Phosphorus 39 mg.

Cranberry Cabbage

This is a great holiday recipe. I especially recommend it for Thanksgiving when some favorites, such as yams, are limited.

6	c shredded red cabbage
1	can whole berry cranberry sauce
1	T lemon juice

In a large saucepan, heat cranberry sauce and lemon juice; bring to a boil. Add cabbage and simmer on low heat until the cabbage is tender and flavors have blended; about 1 hour. Makes 6 servings.

Notes: Per serving: Calories 102, Carbohydrates 25 g, Protein 2 g, Fat 0 g, Sodium 26 mg, Potassium 225 mg, Phosphorus 46 mg.

Mock French Fries

(Oven-fried zucchini with crunch Parmesan crust)

1	T olive oil
¼	c fine breadcrumbs
⅓	c Parmesan cheese
½	tsp dried rosemary
½	tsp crumbled cayenne
	black pepper to taste
1	large egg
4	small green or golden zucchini squash

Preheat over to 400º F. Lightly grease a heavy baking sheet with olive oil (or use spray olive oil). In a shallow dish, combine breadcrumbs, rosemary, cayenne, and black pepper. Mix well. In a second dish, lightly beat the egg. Trim the ends of the squash, and cut each squash lengthwise. Lay the halves flat and cut in half again, then cut the strips in half crosswise. Dredge each piece first in the egg and then in the Parmesan crumb mixture. Bake for 15 minutes or until light brown and crunchy. Makes 8 servings.

Notes: Per serving: Calories 41, Carbohydrates 3 g, Protein 3 g, Fat 2 g, Sodium 100 mg, Potassium 39 mg, Phosphorus 55 mg.

Quinoa Pilaf With Pine Nuts

½   c quinoa

1   c homemade chicken broth (page 45)

2   tsp olive oil

½   large onion, chopped

2   T pine nuts toasted in a dry heat skillet for 2 minutes

2   T fresh parsley, chopped

Bring quinoa and broth to a boil in medium saucepan. Reduce heat to low, cover and cook until quinoa absorbs the liquid, about 15 minutes. Heat oil in a large skillet over medium heat, add onion, and stir occasionally until the onion begins to brown, about 5 minutes. When quinoa is done, fluff with a fork and transfer to a serving bowl. Stir in onion, toasted pine nuts, and parsley, season with pepper to taste. Serves 4.

Notes: Per serving: Calories 172, Carbohydrates 15 g, Protein 4 g, Fat 1 g, Potassium 175 mg, Phosphorus 104 mg.

Rice With Mushrooms

3   c water (less if you want sticky rice)

1½ c uncooked brown or white rice

¾   c mushrooms (white button, cremini, or shiitake), chopped

2   T olive oil

3   cloves garlic, crushed

       pepper to taste

       fresh parsley to taste

Rinse the rice and place the water and rice in a pot. When the water boils, cover the pot and lower the heat to med-low. Cook the rice 25 minutes until all water is absorbed and the rice is done (brown rice takes longer to cook). Meanwhile, heat the olive oil in a skillet, add the garlic and cook 1-2 minutes. Add the chopped mushrooms to the skillet and sauté for 3 minutes. Season with pepper, add the mushrooms to the cooked rice, add parsley and toss to blend. Serves 6.

Mushrooms are a great source of Vitamin D, a wonder vitamin, which helps our body in many ways.

Notes: Per serving: Calories 160, Carbohydrates 27 g, Protein 2 g, Fat 2 g, Sodium 1 mg, Potassium 70 mg, Phosphorus 44 mg.

Curry Style Rice

1	c rice
1	small apple, peeled, cored, and finely chopped
2	T olive oil
½	c onion, chopped
2	cloves garlic, minced
1	T curry powder
½	bay leaf
1½	c homemade chicken broth (page 45)
1	T butter

Measure rice and set aside. Heat 2 T olive oil in a large skillet. Add the onion and garlic, and cook until the onion softens. Add the apple and curry powder; stir. Add the rice, bay leaf, and chicken broth. Cover and cook 17 minutes over medium low heat. Add 1 T butter to rice. Fluff with a fork and serve. Makes 4 servings.

The fresh spices in this recipe are safe for the CKD diet so feel free to load up on them if you find them to be too mild in some of my recipes.

Notes: Per serving: Calories 102, Carbohydrates 13 g, Protein 2 g, Fat 6 g, Sodium 122 mg, Potassium 90 mg, Phosphorus 19 mg.

Brown Rice And Carrot Pilaf

3   T olive oil

1   onion, finely chopped

1   c carrots, finely shredded

1   c brown rice

2½   c vegetable consommé (page 44)

½   c parsley, chopped

Heat olive oil in 2-quart saucepan over medium high heat. Add onions and carrots and cook until onion softens, about 5 minutes. Stir in rice, cook until rice browns slightly. Add vegetable stock, cover and simmer on low heat until rice is tender and liquid is absorbed, about 45 minutes. Stir in parsley. Makes 6 servings ½ c each.

Notes: Per serving: Calories 192, Carbohydrates 28 g, Protein 3 g, Sodium 8 mg, Phosphorus 101 mg, Potassium 186 mg.

Herbed Rice

½	tsp paprika
¼	tsp ground red pepper
¼	tsp black pepper
¼	tsp dry mustard
¼	tsp dried whole thyme
¼	tsp dried whole basil
1	T olive oil
½	c onion, chopped
½	c celery, chopped
½	c green pepper, chopped
1	garlic clove, minced
⅔	c uncooked long grain rice
1	c water

Combine first 6 ingredients (paprika through basil) in a small bowl, mix and set aside. Heat olive oil in a large saucepan. Add onion, celery, green pepper, and garlic to the saucepan and sauté until vegetables are crisp-tender. Stir in rice, and sauté until lightly browned. Stir in reserve seasoning mixture, add water and bring to a boil. Cover, reduce heat to low and simmer for 20 minutes or until liquid is absorbed. Makes 6 servings.

Notes: Per serving: Calories 110, Carbohydrates 20 g, Fat 3 g, Protein 2 g, Sodium 13 mg, Phosphorus 39 mg, Potassium 109 mg.

Byzantine Pilaf

¾   tsp allspice

½   tsp ground cumin

½   tsp ground cardamom

1   T olive oil

1   T butter

1   c onion, chopped

2   cloves garlic, minced

4   medium carrots, peeled, cut, and diced

1½ c long grain white rice

3½ c homemade chicken broth (page 46) or
low sodium store-bought broth

¾   c dried cranberries

Mix allspice, cumin, and cardamom in a small bowl, and set aside. Heat olive oil and butter in a large skillet over low heat, add the onion and cook stirring occasionally until slightly wilted, about 5 minutes. Add the garlic and carrots and cook 5 minutes longer. Add the spice mixture and cook for 1 minute, stirring constantly. Add the rice and cook for 1 minute, stirring constantly. Stir in the chicken broth and cranberries. Increase the heat to medium-high and bring to a boil. Reduce the heat, cover the pot, and cook on low heat until the liquid is absorbed and rice is tender, about 15 minutes. Serves 6.

Notes: Per serving: Calories 272, Carbohydrates 45 g, Protein 9 g, Fat 7 g, Sodium 54 mg, Potassium 200 mg, Phosphorus 128 mg.

Wild Rice With Cranberries

This recipe goes well with roasted chicken. This recipe can also be used as stuffing for acorn squash or Cornish Game Hens.

¼	c dried cranberries
¼	c slivered almonds
¼	c brown sugar
2	c cooked wild rice (cook according to package instructions)
1	c cooked brown rice
½	c celery, sliced
2	T red wine vinegar
1	tsp grated orange peel
⅓	c apple juice

Soak cranberries in hot water for 10 minutes. After, in a medium nonstick skillet, cook cranberries, almonds, and sugar over medium heat, stirring until sugar melts and coats the almonds, almost 3 minutes. Stir in wild rice, brown rice, celery, wine vinegar, grated orange peel, and apple juice. Cook until heated through, about 6 minutes, stirring frequently. Serves 6.

Notes: Per serving: Calories 105, Carbohydrates 24 g, Protein 2 g, Fat 0 g, Sodium 15 mg, Potassium 146 mg, Phosphorus 93 mg.

Garlic Cheese Grits

This recipe is very high in calories. I intend it for those looking to prevent weight loss or trying to gain weight.

4	c water
1	garlic clove, mashed
1	c quick grits
¼	c butter
½	c cheddar cheese, shredded
1	tsp Worcestershire sauce
3	eggs
	paprika to taste
½	c whole milk
	hot sauce to taste

Preheat oven to 300ºF. Bring 4 cups of water to a boil. Add garlic and grits, cook according to the package directions. Add the butter and ¾ of the cheese. In another bowl, beat the eggs and milk, and then add them to the grits mixture. Spray a casserole dish with nonstick spray and pour in grits mixture. Cover and bake at 300ºF for 1 hour. Uncover and sprinkle with remaining cheese. Bake another 15 minutes. Top with paprika and hot sauce to taste. Serving size ¾ c.

Notes: Per serving: Calories 350, Protein 14.9 g, Fat 22 g, Carbohydrates 17.5 mg, Sodium 405 mg, Potassium 116 mg, Phosphorus 279 mg.

Couscous

This cross between rice and pasta is one of my favorite grains. In this case the chicken soup gives the couscous flavor, but you can also use vegetable broth, garlic, and scallions.

1⅓ c couscous (plain Moroccan pasta)
1¾ c homemade chicken stock (page 45)
1   T olive oil

Heat the chicken broth on the stove in a 2-quart pot. When it comes to a boil add the couscous and olive oil. Take off the heat and let sit for 10 minutes until the liquid is absorbed. Fluff with a fork and enjoy. Makes 4 1 cup servings.

Notes: Per serving: Calories 280, Carbohydrates 51 g, Fat 5 g, Protein 10 g, Sodium 23 mg, Phosphorus 128 mg, Potassium 210 mg.

Scrumptious Asparagus

2   lbs Asparagus slender stalks with bottoms removed

2   T olive oil

3   garlic cloves, finely chopped

¼   c homemade chicken stock (page 45)

1   slice ginger (optional)

Warm olive in a heavy frying pan. Add the asparagus (you may also opt to add fresh sliced ginger for an Asian flavor). Stir-fry for 2 minutes. Add garlic and continue cooking for another minute. Add ¼ c chicken stock. Cover pan, reduce heat, and cook until asparagus is tender, about 5 minutes. Serving size is approximately ½ c.

Notes: Per serving: Calories 81, Carbohydrates 4 g, Protein 2 g, fat 6 g, Sodium 2 mg, Phosphorus 43 mg, Potassium 197 mg.

Braised Red Cabbage

1   T olive oil

1   c onion, chopped

1¼   lbs red cabbage, shredded

1   golden delicious apple, peeled and thinly sliced

1   T brown sugar

1   T red wine vinegar

⅛   tsp black pepper

1   c warm water

Heat olive oil in a large skillet. Add the onion and sauté for 1 minute. Add the cabbage and apple; cook, stirring occasionally, for 5 minutes. In a bowl, combine pepper, brown sugar, water, and vinegar. Add this to the cabbage mixture and cook covered for 30 minutes over low heat. Can be served hot or cold. Makes 6 generous servings.

Notes: Per serving: Calories 74, Carbohydrates 13 g, Fat 3 g, Protein 2 g, Phosphorus 51 mg, Sodium 12 mg, Potassium 268 mg.

Pineapple Carrots

2	c carrots cut into thin stalks or baby carrots
6	oz pineapple juice
⅛	tsp nutmeg
¾	tsp cinnamon

Combine all the ingredients in a medium saucepan. Bring the mixture to a boil, reduce the heat and cover the pan, simmer for about 10 minutes or until the carrots are tender-crisp. Makes 3 servings.

Notes: Per serving: Calories 39, Carbohydrates 9 g, Protein 1 g, Fat 0, Sodium 23 mg, Phosphorus 30 mg, Potassium 236 mg.

Cauliflower With Butter Crumb Topping

2   qt water

2   c cauliflower florets

2   T salted butter

2   T seasoned breadcrumbs

Boil 2 qt water. Add cauliflower and cook uncovered for 5 minutes. Meanwhile, melt butter in saucepan, and add breadcrumbs. When cauliflower is tender take it off the stove and drain the water. Put the cauliflower into the butter and bread-crumb mixture and stir to cover the cauliflower well. Makes 4 servings.

Notes: Per serving: Calories 77, Carbohydrates 5 g, Protein 2 g, Fat 5 g, Potassium 161 mg, Phosphorus 29 mg, Sodium 103 mg.

Green Beans With Garlic And Basil

2   c water

1½   lbs green beans, trimmed

2   T olive oil

2   garlic cloves, chopped

2   T fresh basil, finely chopped

¼   tsp black pepper

Bring a large saucepan ¾-full of water to a boil. Add the beans and boil until barely tender, and resistant to the bite, 3-4 minutes. Drain well. In a heavy frying pan over medium heat warm the olive oil. When the oil is hat add the beans and stir often until they begin to brown slightly, about 3 minutes. Add the garlic and basil and toss for 30 seconds. Remove from heat and add black pepper to taste. Makes 6 servings.

Notes: Per serving: Calories 58, Carbohydrates 4 g, Fat 4 g, Protein 2 g, Phosphorus 33 mg, Potassium 124 mg, Sodium 3 mg.

Green Beans With Roasted Onions

Vegetable oil spray

6   onions, peeled and cut into 12-14 wedges

3   T butter

1   c homemade chicken broth (page 45)

1½   T sugar

1   T red wine vinegar

1½   lb Green beans, trimmed

¼   tsp black pepper

Preheat oven to 450ºF. Spray a large heavy baking sheet with vegetable oil spray. Arrange onions in a single layer on sheet. Dot the onions with 1 ½ T butter, and season with black pepper. Bake until the onions are brown, about 30 minutes. Meanwhile, boil broth in a saucepan until reduced to ¼ c., about 6 minutes. Add sugar and vinegar and whisk until sugar dissolves and mixture returns to a boil. Add onions to sauce, reduce heat to medium low. Simmer 5 minutes. Season mixture with pepper. The sauce can be prepared 1 day in advance. Cook green beans in a large pot of boiling water until crisp-tender, about 5 minutes. Drain well. Return beans to the same pot and add the rest of the butter, toss to coat. Add the beans to a plate and top with onion mixture. Makes 6 servings.

Notes: Per serving: Calories 130, Carbohydrates 16 g, Fat 3 g, Protein 4 g, Sodium 55 mg, Phosphorus 83 mg, Potassium 246 mg.

Herbed Baby Vegetables

1½ tsp olive oil

2 cloves garlic, crushed

½ tsp dried whole thyme

½ tsp dried rosemary, crushed

⅔ lb baby eggplant, quartered

⅔ lb baby zucchini, quartered

2 tsp fresh parsley

Coat a large nonstick skillet with cooking spray; add the oil and heat over medium heat until hot. Add garlic, thyme, rosemary, and black pepper. Sauté 1 minute. Add the remaining ingredients and sauté 5 minutes until crisp-tender, stirring occasionally. Serves 8.

Notes: Per serving: Calories 35, Carbohydrates 4 g, Fat 2 g, Protein 1 g, Sodium 19 mg, Phosphorus 45 mg, Potassium 260 mg.

Zucchini And Carrots
A La Menthe

3   carrots, peeled and cut into quarter inch rounds

2   zucchini, ends trimmed

2   T olive oil

2   tsp mint, finely chopped

2   tsp parsley, chopped

    pepper to taste

Peel carrots and cut into quarter inch rounds, trim ends from the zucchini and cut into quarter inch rounds. Set aside. Heat olive oil in a heavy skillet and then add the carrots and pepper. Cook covered about 3-5 minutes until half cooked. Add the zucchini and cover. Shake skillet occasionally, cook 4-5 minutes or until all the vegetables are crisp-tender. Sprinkle with pepper, mint, and parsley. Serves 4.

Notes: Per serving: Calories 45, Carbohydrates 4 g, Protein 0 g, Fat 2 g, Sodium 5 mg, Potassium 105 mg, Phosphorus 15 mg.

Main Dishes

Frozen Entrees Comparison

Entrees falling within CKD guidelines at time of publication with available information. These are acceptable to eat.

Lean Cuisine Chicken Enchilada Suiza

Kashi Red Curry Chicken

Kashi Black Bean Mango

Kashi Mayan Harvest Bake

Amy's Organic Asian Noodle Stir Fry

Amy's Organic Bean and Rice Burrito

Amy's Organic Black Bean Enchilada

Amy's Organic Breakfast Burrito

Amy's Organic Country Vegetable Pie

Amy's Organic Mexican Casserole Bowl

Amy's Organic Soy Cheese Pizza

Amy's Organic Thai Stir Fry

Amy's Organic Light in Sodium Black Bean Enchilada

Amy's Organic light in Sodium Vegetable Lasagna

Amy's Organic Light in Sodium Mexican Casserole Bowl

(continued)

I am a big fan of home cooking and minimizing fast food and convenience foods, but in life there are times that they meet a need. I am offering you this information so that when the need arises you have some options. In prepared foods, the potassium and phosphorus are mostly found in the foods' additives and not in the foods themselves. The additives are absorbed rapidly into the bloodstream and have been shown to increase the progression of kidney disease.

Potassium and phosphorus are not mandated to be on the label, so many food manufacturers do not offer this information. At this time I am lacking information for most Weight Watchers and Healthy Choice Entrees, but by looking at their list of food additives I am not sure they are the best for CKD patients.

Frozen entrees not meeting CKD guidelines

    Lean Cuisine Chicken and Vegetables with Vermicelli
    Kashi Sweet and Sour Chicken
    Kashi Tuscan Vegetable Bake
    Amy's Organic Brown Rice Vegetable Bowl
    Amy's Organic Chili and Cornbread Whole Meal
    Amy's Organic Shepherd's Pie
    Amy's Organic Tofu Vegetable Lasagna
    Amy's Organic Light in Sodium Veggie Loaf

Dining Out Guide

(Acceptable Options at Various Restaurants)

Arby's: Martha's Vineyard salad with raspberry vinaigrette

Bruegger's all bagels are fine

Burger King: Garden Salad (no chicken) with dressing

Domino's: 12" or 14" cheese, veggie pizza, 1 slice

KFC: Extra crispy whole wing or drumstick, corn, coleslaw, house salad

McDonald's: Side salad, fruit salad, apple dippers

Panera: Bagels, cheese artisan pastry, apple artisan pastry, croissant, Caesar salad with apple, fandango salad with apple or baguette

Papa John's: cheese pizza, 1 slice

Pizza Hut: cheese pizza, 1 slice

Subway: 6" Veggie Delight, Tuna deli

Fast food restaurants use a lot of additives, which make many of their meals too high in potassium and phosphorus. The food additives have also been shown to accelerate kidney disease. You may be looking at this list thinking, "there is not much to choose from," and you are right. Chain restaurants usually have a central kitchen and send their food and sauce long distances. They use a large quantity of food additives to make the food shelf stable, and to enhance flavors.

(continued)

These food additives are harmful and accelerate kidney disease, so I try to minimize them in your diet.

My advice to you is that if you do not want to cook all the time and want a special meal out, find Mom and Pop restaurants, where Mama is serving you fresh homemade meals. This type of restaurant uses basic, healthy food ingredients, and because the food does not have to live on the shelf for months there are not the same concentration of food additives. You can select basic fish and chicken meals with vegetables from the list. Homemade soups are acceptable options; however, the commercial ones are especially loaded with food additives. I worry less about the sodium than the potassium and phosphorus laden food additives. The amount of potassium and phosphorus they add to the meal is more than 10 times the amount you might possibly get from fresh unprocessed foods. Your sodium budget is 2000-2200 mg per day so keep that in mind as well when dining out.

Pizza Margherita

1	12 oz Boboli pizza crust or Trader Joe's pizza dough
1½	tsp olive oil, divided
2	garlic cloves, minced
2	plum tomatoes, very thinly sliced
4	oz shredded fresh mozzarella cheese
1	tsp balsamic vinegar
½	c fresh basil, thinly sliced
	black pepper to taste

Preheat oven according to package directions. Spread the minced garlic cloves on top of the Boboli crust and cover the crust with 1 tsp olive oil. Blot out excess moisture from tomato slices and arrange them on the crust leaving a slight border. Sprinkle the pizza evenly with cheese. Bake for 12 minutes or until the cheese melts and the crust is golden. Combine ½ tsp olive oil and 1 tsp balsamic vinegar to make balsamic vinaigrette. Stir with a whisk. Sprinkle pizza evenly with fresh basil and black pepper, and drizzle with the balsamic vinaigrette. Cut pizza into four slices.

Notes: Per serving: Calories 146, Carbohydrates 11 g, Protein 7 g, Fat 8 g, Sodium 202 mg, Potassium 123 mg, Phosphorus 126 mg. Use Trader Joe's pizza dough or other fresh dough to reduce sodium.

Barbecue Chicken Pizza

2	T olive oil
2	large boneless chicken breasts
½	c hickory style BBQ sauce
7	oz smoked Gouda cheese
1	12 oz Boboli pizza crust or Trader Joe's pizza dough
¾	c red onions, sliced
3	green onions, chopped
	fresh cilantro to taste
	black pepper to taste

Preheat oven to 450ºF. Heat olive oil in a heavy skillet over medium high heat. Season chicken with pepper and add to skillet, cook until just cooked through about 5 minutes per side. Transfer chicken to plate and rest 5 minutes. Cut chicken crosswise into 1/3 inch slices. Transfer chicken to a bowl and toss with ¼ c barbecue sauce. Spread half the cheese on the Boboli, and evenly arrange the chicken slices. Add remaining barbecue sauce on top. Sprinkle red onion over the chicken top with remaining cheese and green onion. Bake until bottom of crust is crisp and cheese has melted, about 14 minutes. Let stand 5 minutes, sprinkle with cilantro and serve. Serves 6.

Due to the high sodium content in the pizza I consider it a special occasion meal. You can make your own barbecue sauce to greatly reduce the sodium content. I also suggest using fresh dough such as Trader Joe's or your own dough to reduce the sodium content and tastes much better.

Notes: Per serving: Calories 356, Carbohydrates 21 g, Protein 26 g, Fat 15 g, Sodium 620 mg, Potassium 323 mg, Phosphorus 364 mg.

Asian Style Chicken Pizza

1	12 oz Boboli pizza crust or fresh dough or Trader Joe's fresh pizza dough (follow rolling directions)
1	c rice vinegar
⅓	c brown sugar
3	T low sodium soy sauce
2	T water
1	T fresh ginger, peeled and minced
1½	T peanut butter
¾	tsp crushed red pepper
4	garlic cloves, minced
	cooking spray
½	lb skinless, boneless chicken breast cut into bite-sized pieces
2	oz reduced fat reduced sodium Swiss cheese such as Alpine Lace
1	oz shredded part skim Mozzarella cheese
¼	c green onions, chopped
	cilantro to taste

Preheat oven to 500ºF. Heat nonstick skillet coated with cooking spray over medium heat; add chicken and sauté 2 minutes. Remove chicken from the pan. Mix vinegar, brown sugar, soy sauce, water, fresh ginger, peanut butter, red pepper, and garlic.

Add to the skillet and bring to a boil over medium high heat. Cook 6 minutes until slightly thickened.

(continued)

Return chicken to pan, cook 1 minute per side. Sprinkle cheeses over prepared crust, leaving a ½ inch border, and top pizza crust with chicken mixture. Bake at 500ºF for 12 minutes directly on the oven rack. Sprinkle with green onions and cilantro. Serves 6.

This meal is much higher in sodium than I usually strive for, but it is still far lower in sodium than frozen or restaurant pizza. Use fresh dough or Trader Joe's to reduce sodium content. Follow directions on dough pkg

Notes: Per serving: Calories 376, Carbohydrates 43 g, Protein 28 g, Fat 10 g, Sodium 673 mg, Potassium 370 mg, Phosphorus 288 mg.

Pizza With Caramelized Onions and Gorgonzola Cheese

2	tsp olive oil
12	c onion, thinly sliced
3	cloves garlic, minced
2	tsp chopped fresh rosemary or ½ tsp dried rosemary
	black pepper to taste
12	inch Boboli pizza crust or Trader Joe's fresh dough
2	oz Gorgonzola cheese
1	c raw arugula
	balsamic vinaigrette drizzle or balsamic vinegar spray

Preheat oven to 500ºF. Heat oil in a skillet, add onion, and sauté 5 minutes. Stir in half of the rosemary and black pepper to taste. Continue cooking 15 minutes or until the onion is deep golden brown, stirring frequently. Top Boboli with the cooked onion, bake for 10 minutes, add the cheese and bake for an additional 3 minutes. Remove from oven, top with the remainder rosemary and arugula. Spray the arugula lightly with the balsamic or drizzle a thin layer of balsamic vinaigrette. Serves 4.

Notes: Per serving: Calories 186, Carbohydrates 27 g, Protein 7 g, Fat 6 g, Sodium 139 mg, Potassium 379 mg, Phosphorus 122 mg.

Chicken Chilaquiles

2	c skinless, boneless chicken breast, cooked
½	c green onions, chopped
2	oz jalapeno Monterey Jack cheese, coarsely shredded, divided
2	T grated Parmesan cheese
1	tsp chili powder
	black pepper to taste
¾	c low fat milk
¼	c fresh cilantro
8	oz salsa verde
10	corn tortillas
	cooking spray

Preheat oven to 375ºF. Combine chicken, green onion, ¼ c Monterey Jack cheese, Parmesan cheese, chili powder, and pepper in a bowl. Place milk, cilantro, and Salsa Verde in a food processor or blender and process until smooth. Wrap tortillas in a paper towel and microwave 1 minute until soft and warm. Spray 11x7 glass baking dish with vegetable cooking spray. Pour 1/3 Salsa Verde mixture in the bottom of a dish. Arrange 4 corn tortillas in dish and top with half the chicken mixture, repeat layer with remaining tortillas and chicken mixture ending with tortillas.

Pour remaining SalsaVerde mixture over the tortillas and sprinkle with remaining ¼ c Monterey Jack cheese. Bake at 375ºF. Cheese should be bubbling. Serves 4.

Notes: Per serving: Calories 311, Carbohydrates 32 g, Protein 24 g, Fat 9 g, Sodium 350 mg, Potassium 295 mg, Phosphorus 430 mg.

Moo Shoo Chicken In Tortillas

2	T peanut oil
2	boneless chicken breasts, sliced into thin long pieces
1	tsp cornstarch
2	cloves garlic, peeled and minced
2	c broccoli flowerets
1	c mushrooms, sliced
10	oz coleslaw mix
2	T prepared Teriyaki sauce
½	c spring onions or scallions, chopped
8	flour tortillas
1	T Hoisin sauce

Heat the 1 T peanut oil in a deep skillet. Toss the chicken with cornstarch in a bowl. Add chicken to skillet and cook until beginning to brown, about 3-4 minutes. Transfer to a plate. Add remaining oil to the skillet and add garlic, cook 5 minutes. Add vegetables and Teriyaki sauce. Cook stirring frequently until vegetables are tender-crisp, 5-7 minutes. Return chicken to skillet and cook 1 minute. Wrap tortillas in a paper towel and microwave for 1 minute until soft and warm. To serve, spread Hoisin sauce on the tortilla and 1/8 of the chicken and vegetable mixture. Wrap them up and the tortillas are ready to serve. Serves 4; 2 tortillas each.

Hoisin sauce is now found in most supermarkets in their ethnic aisles. It is a little bit higher in sodium than what I usually try to give you, but it has just a fraction of the sodium you would get at a restaurant and it does not contain MSG.

Notes: Per serving: Calories 248, Protein 12 g, Carbohydrates 40 g, Fat 5 g, Sodium 642 mg, Potassium 288 mg, Phosphorus 169 mg.

Chicken Rogan Josh

The yogurt marinade makes this chicken dish exceptionally tender and the spices make your taste buds sing.

3	lbs boneless chicken pieces
⅛	tsp black pepper
2	c plain non-fat yogurt
1	large onion, finely chopped
5	cloves garlic, minced
¼	c fresh ginger, minced
1	tsp ground coriander
1	tsp ground cardamom
½	tsp ground cloves
½	tsp ground turmeric
2	T butter
2	T vegetable oil
6	c homemade chicken broth (page 45)
¼	c coarsely chopped fresh cilantro leaves

Rinse the chicken and pat dry. Place the chicken in a bowl and add yogurt and pepper. Coat the chicken well and let marinate at room temperature for 1 hour.

Combine the onion, garlic, ginger, coriander, cardamom, cloves, and turmeric in a food processor or blender. Pulse on and off to combine until a smooth paste is formed. Heat the butter and oil in a large skillet over low heat. Add the onion and spice puree and cook stirring over medium heat for 5 minutes. Add the marinated chicken and yogurt. Add enough chicken broth to cover the chicken and bring to a simmer. Reduce heat to low and stir well, cook covered until the chicken is cooked through, about 45 minutes. Stir in cilantro and serve over rice.

Notes: Per serving: Without the rice, Calories 206, Carbohydrates 4 g, Protein 25 g, Fat 10 g, Sodium 96 mg, Potassium 359 mg, Phosphorus 295 mg.

Chicken Tikka

1	2" piece fresh ginger, peeled and coarsely chopped
6	cloves garlic, coarsely chopped
4	T lemon juice
1	c plain non-fat yogurt
2	T vegetable oil
2	tsp chili powder
4	whole boneless skinless chicken breasts halved
3	medium onions, halved and slivered
1	tsp ground cumin
⅛	tsp ground turmeric
2	T fresh parsley

Place the ginger, garlic, 2 T lemon juice, and ¼ c yogurt in a food processor or blender and puree until smooth. Scrape the puree into a bowl and add the remaining ¾ c yogurt and chili powder, stir well. Cut each halved chicken breast crosswise and into 3 pieces and add the chicken to the yogurt mixture and toss to coat. Marinate at room temperature for 1 hour. Meanwhile, place the onions in a large bowl and add 2 T lemon juice, 2 T vegetable oil, cumin, and turmeric, set aside. 15 minutes before the chicken has finished marinating, preheat the broiler or grill.

Spread the onions in a single layer on a baking sheet and broil until they are golden, about 10 minutes. Remove the chicken pieces from the marinade with a fork and broil in small batches in a large cast iron skillet over medium high heat or grill on an outdoor grill. Divide the onions evenly among the 6 dinner plates, top with chicken pieces and sprinkle with chopped parsley. Goes well with rice. Serves 6.

Notes: Per serving without the rice, Calories 109, Carbohydrates 3 g, Fat 1 g, Protein 21 g, Sodium 74 mg, Potassium 287 mg, Phosphorus 198 mg.

Lemon-Herb Roasted Chicken

The entire family will come running when the aroma of the cooking chicken spreads through the house.

3	T olive oil
2	T chopped fresh rosemary or 2 tsp dried rosemary
2	T chopped fresh thyme or 2 tsp dried thyme
5	garlic cloves, minced
1½	tsp lemon peel, finely chopped
6	lb roasting chicken
	black pepper to taste

Combine olive oil, rosemary, thyme, garlic, and lemon peel in a small bowl and stir to blend. Season with black pepper. Can be prepared 1-2 days ahead of time. Preheat oven to 450°F. Rinse the chicken and pat dry. Slide hand under the skin of the chicken breast to loosen the skin from the meat. Bring herbed oil to room temperature and rub herbed oil under the skin and all over the chicken. Sprinkle additional pepper, rosemary, and thyme all over the chicken. Place in a large roasting pan. Roast 20 minutes. Reduce oven temperature to 375°F and roast an additional 1 hour 15 minutes. Serving size is 3 oz chicken meat.

Notes: Per 3 oz serving, Calories 260, Protein 23.6 g, Fat 12 g, Carbohydrates 1 g, Sodium 71 mg, Potassium 370 mg, Phosphorus 220 mg.

Chicken Parisienne

4	chicken breasts
½	c onions, sliced
¼	c green pepper, sliced
1	c mushrooms, sliced
¾	c orange juice
½	c water
3	T sherry
1	T orange zest
1	T brown sugar
1	T flour
2	tsp parsley
¼	tsp black pepper

Place chicken in baking dish. Put onions, green pepper, and mushrooms over the chicken. In a saucepan, combine orange juice, water, sherry, orange zest, brown sugar, flour, dried parsley, and black pepper. Cook until thickened. Pour over the chicken. Bake at 375°F for 1 hour, and baste occasionally. Serving size is 1 medium chicken breast.

Notes: Per serving, Calories 205, Protein 26 g, Fat 3.4 g, Carbohydrates 14 g, Sodium 154 mg, Potassium 340 mg, Phosphorus 238 mg.

Orange Chicken

This is a fast and easy dish that tastes as if you spent the whole day in the kitchen.

½	c orange juice
¼	c brown sugar
¼	c honey
1	T prepared yellow mustard
1	c corn flakes crumbs
¼	tsp black pepper
1	lb chicken cut up, skin removed

Combine orange juice, brown sugar, honey, and mustard in a saucepan over medium heat. Simmer for 5 minutes and let cool. Combine corn flakes and pepper. Dip the chicken in the cooled sauce and roll in crumb mixture to coat evenly. Place in a single layer on greased or foil lined baking pan. Bake at 350°F for 1 hour. Do not turn the chicken during baking. Serves 6.

Notes: Per serving: Calories 230, Protein 18 g, Fat 3 g, Carbohydrates 42 g, Sodium 313 mg, Potassium 160 mg, Phosphorus 121 mg.

Thai Rice Noodles With Chicken

¼ c lime juice, divided

2 boneless, skinless chicken breasts cut into ¼" cubes

8 oz thick rice noodles

1 T brown sugar

1 T water

½ T fish sauce

½ T low sodium soy sauce

1½ tsp chili paste with garlic

4 tsp vegetable oil, divided

3 T green onions, sliced

1 tsp fresh ginger, grated

½ c torn fresh basil

¼ c lemongrass, thinly sliced

¼ c shallots, vertically sliced

Combine 2 T lime juice and chicken in a bowl, let stand 15 minutes. Soak noodles in hot water 15 minutes until soft, but still chewy; drain. Combine 2 T lime juice, sugar, fish sauce, soy sauce, and chili sauce, and set mixture aside. Heat 1 T vegetable oil in a large skillet over medium heat and swirl to coat. Remove chicken from juice and add to pan. Stir-fry 4 minutes, and then transfer to large bowl. Add 1 T oil to the pan, add green onions and ginger, and stir-fry for 45 seconds or until just golden and fragrant. Add noodles and cook 30 seconds, tossing well. Place 1 ¼ c noodle mixture on each of the 4 plates. Top with 2 T basil leaves and 1 T lemongrass, and 1 T shallots. Makes 4 servings.

(continued)

This meal is higher in salt than some of my other recipes, but it a large improvement over what you might get if you ate out at a restaurant. The ingredients are carried by most large grocery stores in their "ethnic" aisles.

Notes: Per serving: Calories 385, Carbohydrates 54 g, Protein 26 g, Fat 5 g, Sodium 420 mg, Potassium 348 mg, Phosphorus 291 mg.

French Bistro Chicken

This is a family favorite! The fragrant juices go well on top of rice accompanied by a fresh garden salad.

1	lb chicken, legs, thighs, and breast skin removed
3	T olive oil
3	T balsamic vinegar
½	c shallots, chopped
2	tsp dried thyme
2	tsp dried rosemary
½	tsp black pepper

Rinse and pat the chicken pieces dry. Pour olive oil in a 12x8 inch-baking dish. Place chicken in the dish and lightly coat all surfaces with the oil. Sprinkle with vinegar and shallots; sprinkle half the herbs over the chicken. Roast the chicken in a preheated oven at 400°F, uncovered for 20 minutes. Turn the chicken and sprinkle the remaining herbs over the chicken. Increase the oven temperature to 425°F and roast an additional 20 minutes. Serves 4-5.

Notes: Per serving: Calories 235, Carbohydrates 5 g, Protein 27 g, Fat 12 g, Sodium 77 mg, Phosphorus 238 mg, Potassium 265 mg.

Oven "Fried" Chicken

This is a delicious and simple recipe that tastes great served hot or cold in a garden salad.

6	chicken legs and thighs, without skin
1	c milk
½	c plain breadcrumbs or crumbled corn flakes
⅓	c Parmesan cheese, grated
1	T dried parsley flakes, crumbled
¼	tsp black pepper
	vegetable cooking spray

Place the chicken pieces in a shallow bowl and cover them with milk. Let the chicken soak for 15 minutes or longer. In a shallow bowl, combine the breadcrumbs or corn flakes, cheese, parsley flakes, and pepper. One by one dip the soaked chicken pieces in the breading mixture, coating well on all sides. Set the coated chicken on a greased baking sheet with a nonstick surface. Spray the chicken pieces with vegetable oil spray. Bake the chicken in a preheated oven at 375ºF for about 45 minutes. Makes 6 servings.

Notes: Per serving: Calories 150, Carbohydrates 6 g, Protein 21 g, Fat 3 g, Sodium 212 mg, Phosphorus 214 mg, Potassium 239 mg.

Chicken Lo Mein

4	c water
12	oz pasta, dry and uncooked
2	T Worcestershire sauce
1	T low sodium soy sauce
1	T cooking sherry
2	T olive oil, divided
3	scallions, thinly sliced
3	garlic cloves, minced
1	sweet red pepper, cut into thin strips
1	c homemade broth (any type)
1	c cooked chicken

Cook noodles in a large pot of boiling water until they are just short of being done (al dente); drain the noodles. In a small bowl combine Worcestershire sauce, soy sauce, and sherry; set aside. In a large skillet heat 1 tablespoon of olive oil and stir-fry the scallions, garlic, and red pepper for 1 minute. Add the cabbage, and stir-fry the vegetables for another minute. Add the chicken and stir-fry another minute. Transfer the mixture to a bowl. Heat the remaining oil over high heat; add the noodles and let them brown for 2 minutes. Reduce the heat and add the broth. Stir well.

Add the vegetable mixture and Worcestershire sauce mixture to the noodles. Toss and heat through for 1 minute. Sprinkle with hot pepper oil if desired. Makes 4 servings.

Notes: per serving: Calories 468, Carbohydrates 69 g, Protein 24 g, Fat 10 g, Sodium 413 mg, Phosphorus 272 mg, Potassium 357 mg.

Rice With Chicken

This is a great complete meal in one pot.

1	T olive oil
5	oz ground turkey sausage
1½	c uncooked, boneless chicken cut into 1" pieces
8	oz canned whole tomatoes, drained and cut into large pieces
3¼	c homemade chicken broth (page 45)
1	c onion, chopped
½	c green pepper, chopped
3	garlic cloves, crushed
1½	c medium grain white rice, uncooked

Heat olive oil in a 10" skillet. Sauté ground turkey until browned and then transfer to a plate. Sprinkle black pepper on chicken pieces, add chicken to the skillet until browned on all sides, about 5 minutes, transfer to a plate. Sauté the onion and green pepper in the skillet over medium heat until browned, about 3 minutes. Add the garlic, sauté for 1 minute. Stir in the rice until the rice is coated with oil. Stir in the broth, pepper to taste, and heat to boiling. Stir in the reserved turkey meat and chicken. Place the tomatoes on top. Cover and cook over medium heat for 15 minutes or until most of the liquid has been absorbed. Uncover, add the peas and cook covered for 5 more minutes. Uncover and cook over medium heat for 2-5 minutes to cook off any excess moisture. Makes 4, 1 c servings.

Notes: Per serving: Calories 332, Carbohydrates 46, Fat 6 g, Protein 22 g, Sodium 263 mg, Phosphorus 238 mg, Potassium 421 mg.

Terrific Turkey Loaf

2	lbs ground turkey, raw
1	c breadcrumbs
1	c milk
2	eggs, slightly beaten
2	T prepared mustard
3	T ketchup
3	T onion, minced
5	oz cheddar cheese, shredded
	ketchup and cinnamon to taste for topping

Mix all ingredients together except the cheese, ketchup, and cinnamon. Put 1/3 meat mixture in meat loaf pan. Add ½ of the cheddar cheese. Add second layer of meat loaf, and then add the remainder of the cheese. Finally, add the last layer of the meat mixture. Cover top with ketchup and sprinkle with cinnamon. Bake meatloaf at 350°F for 50-60 minutes.

Notes: Per 3 oz serving: Calories 261, Carbohydrates 12 g, Fat 14 g, Protein 22 g, Sodium 367 mg, Phosphorus 259 mg, Potassium 320 mg.

Asian-Inspired
Turkey Meatballs

I admit this recipe is a bit more labor-intensive than others, but the flavor is well worth it. The meatballs can be made ahead and freeze well. Just reheat them in the broth and serve with the sauce on a bed of rice.

1	lb ground turkey
1	T low sodium soy sauce
1	T onion, minced
2	garlic cloves, minced
1	egg
4	c water
2	T low sodium soy sauce
1	T fresh ginger, minced
1	tsp cornstarch
1	T cold water
1	c Asian chicken broth (page 45)

In a medium bowl, combine turkey, 1 T soy sauce, onion, garlic, and egg. Shape the mixture into balls about 1 ½ inch in diameter. Place the meatballs on a tray so they do not touch. In a wide saucepan combine the broth ingredients: water, 2 T soy sauce, and fresh ginger. Bring this to a boil. Add the meatballs one at a time and reduce the heat. Cover the pan and simmer the meatballs for about 30 minutes.

(continued)

Remove the meatballs to a platter and keep warm.

To make the sauce, combine the cornstarch with the cold water in a small saucepan; mix well. Stir warm Asian chicken broth into the saucepan. Bring the sauce to a boil and cook it, stirring until it thickens, about 1 minute. Pour the sauce over the meatballs. Serving size is 4 meatballs.

Notes: Per serving: Calories 193, Carbohydrates 1 g, Fat 11 g, Protein 20 g, Sodium 332 mg, Potassium 288 mg, Phosphorus 208 mg.

Tex-Mex Turkey Tacos

1	c onion, chopped
2	garlic cloves, minced
1	lb ground turkey
1	c frozen whole kernel corn
½	c water
⅛	tsp black pepper
8	oz canned black beans, drained and rinsed
4	oz tomato sauce
1	c white rice, cooked
3	canned chipotle chilies in adobo sauce
10	8" flour tortillas

Heat a large nonstick skillet over medium high heat. Coat the pan with cooking spray. Add onion, garlic, and turkey. Cook 6 minutes or until browned; stirring to crumble the turkey. Stir in corn, water, black pepper, black beans, tomato sauce, cooked rice and chilies. Bring to a boil, reduce heat and simmer 10 minutes. Wrap tortillas in a paper towel and microwave for 30 seconds, until the tortillas are warm and soft. Spoon ½ c turkey mixture into each tortilla and serve. Serving size is 1 taco, and the recipe makes 10 tacos.

Notes: Per serving: Calories 165, Carbohydrates 19 g, Protein 11 g, Fat 4 g, Sodium 328 mg, Potassium 345 mg, Phosphorus 183 mg.

Honey Dijon Salmon

This is a recipe I created after tasting it at the Monocle, a restaurant on Capitol Hill frequented by politicians.

¼	c pineapple juice
12	oz salmon filet
3	T honey
3	T Dijon mustard
3	T spring onions, thinly sliced
¼	c white wine

Soak the salmon filet in pineapple juice in a glass casserole dish for 15 minutes; turning the filet over after 7 minutes. Discard the juice and return the salmon to the glass dish. Combine the honey and mustard, spread this mixture over the salmon filets, and top with the spring onion slices. Broil for 10-12 minutes, basting halfway through and sprinkling with white wine during cooking. Cook until the fish flakes easily. Garnish with lemon slices. Serves 4.

Notes: Per serving: Calories 188, Carbs 15g, Fat 6 g, Protein 18 g, Sodium 170 mg, Potassium 193 mg, Potassium 446 mg.

Broiled Salmon With Dill and Lemon Juice

Fresh dill and lemon juice really bring out the flavor of salmon.

14	oz salmon filets
½	c onions, sliced
2	T olive oil
2	T fresh dill
1	tsp black pepper

Preheat the broiler. Place onion slices on the bottom of the broiler pan and place the salmon on top, skin side down. Spread the olive oil on top of the filet, season with pepper, and sprinkle with lemon juice and dill on top. Broil 12-15 minutes until the fish is opaque. Serves 4.

Notes: Per serving: Calories 250, Carbohydrates 2 g, Protein 20 g, Fat 18g, Sodium 59 mg, Phosphorus 236 mg, Potassium 379 mg.

Chipotle Shrimp Tacos

2	tsp chili powder
1	tsp sugar
½	tsp ground cumin
¼	tsp chipotle chili powder
1½	lb shrimp, peeled and deveined
1	tsp olive oil
8	corn tortillas
2	c iceberg lettuce
1	small avocado, peeled and cut into 16 slices
¾	c salsa verde

Combine chili powder, sugar, cumin, and chipotle chili powder in a large bowl. Add shrimp, tossing to coat. Heat oil in a large skillet, add shrimp to pan and cook 1 to 2 minutes per side until done. Remove from the heat. Heat tortillas between paper towels in the microwave 4 at a time until soft. Arrange 4 shrimp on each tortilla. Top each tortilla with ¼ c lettuce, 2 avocado slices, and 1 ½ T salsa verde. Fold over and serve. Makes 8 tacos, 2 tacos per serving.

If you have been told to limit your potassium severely and you want to decrease the amount in this recipe, omit the avocado slices.

Notes: Per serving: Calories 261, Carbohydrates 31 g, Protein 14 g, Fat 10 g, Sodium 360 mg, Potassium 430 mg, Phosphorus 282 mg.

Fish Tacos With Lime-Cilantro Aioli

Aioli

¼	c green onions, thinly sliced
¼	c fresh cilantro, chopped
3	T fat-free mayonnaise
3	T reduced fat sour cream
1	tsp grated lime rind
1½	tsp lime juice
1	garlic clove, minced

Tacos

1	tsp ground cumin
1	tsp ground coriander
½	tsp ground paprika
¼	tsp ground red pepper
⅛	tsp garlic powder
1½	lb white fish
	cooking spray
8	corn tortillas
2	cups shredded cabbage

Preheat oven to 425ºF. To prepare the aioli combine the first 7 ingredients in a small bowl and set aside. To prepare the tacos, combine cumin, coriander, paprika,

(continued)

red pepper, and garlic powder in a small bowl. Sprinkle the spice mixture on both sides of the fish. Place the fish on a baking sheet coated with cooking spray. Bake at 425°F for 9 minutes or until the fish flakes easily. Place the fish in a bowl and break into large pieces with a fork. Heat tortillas 3 at a time in the microwave for 30-45 seconds or until soft and warm. Divide the fish evenly among the 8 tortillas top each with ¼ c cabbage and 1 T aioli. Makes 8 tacos, 2 tacos per serving.

Most of the potassium in this recipe comes from the fish, which is a low fat, healthy source of protein. Most protein sources; animal, legumes, and soy; are a considerable source of potassium, but protein is essential to everyone's diet so it is calculated in.

Notes: Per serving: Calories 231, Carbohydrates 28 g, Protein 14 g, Fat 7 g, Sodium 199 mg, Potassium 460 mg, Phosphorus 327 mg.

Grilled Grouper
With Salsa Verde

4   6 oz fish fillets (grouper, sea bass, tilapia, sole, cod)

2   T lime juice

2   T fresh garlic, minced

¾   c bottled green salsa

4   T reduced fat sour cream

     additional cilantro for garnish

Drizzle the fish filets with the lime juice, black pepper, and cilantro. Grill 4 minutes on each side or until the fish flakes easily when tested with a fork. Top each fish with sour cream and salsa, garnish with cilantro. Serves 4.

Notes: Per serving: Calories 207, Protein 17 g, Carbohydrates 4 g, Fat 4 g, Sodium 313 mg, Potassium 475 mg, Phosphorus 235 mg.

Baked Fish Ole

Do not pass by this recipe. The ingredients blend together in perfect harmony and taste as if you were eating at the finest restaurant.

1½	lb fresh haddock or other white fish
	vegetable cooking spray
⅓	c salsa
3	T lite mayonnaise
3	T Monterey Jack Cheese with jalapeno peppers, shredded
⅓	tsp pepper

Select a white fish such as Haddock, Orange Roughy, or Sole. Place the fish on a baking sheet coated with vegetable cooking spray. Spray the fish as well. Mix together the salsa, mayonnaise and place on top of the fish; sprinkle the cheese on top. Bake at 400ºF for 15-20 minutes until the fish flakes easily. Serves 4.

Notes: Per serving: Calories 190, Protein 26 g, Carbohydrates 2 g, Fat 8 g, Sodium 360 mg, Potassium 460 mg, Phosphorus 275 mg.

Seafood Cakes
With Mustard Aioli

Sauce

⅓   c light sour cream

7   T fresh parsley, chopped

1   T stone-ground prepared mustard

⅛   tsp black pepper, divided

Seafood Cakes

3   T olive oil, divided

¼   c red onion, finely chopped

¼   c celery, finely chopped

8   oz shrimp, peeled

8   oz lump crab meat, drained

1   oz Parmigiano-Reggiano cheese, freshly grated

2   large egg whites, lightly beaten

1   large egg

1   c Panko breadcrumbs

For the sauce: Combine sour cream, 2 T parsley, mustard, and half the black pepper; stir with a whisk and set aside.

To make the cakes: Head a large nonstick skillet over medium heat. Add 1 tsp olive oil to the pan and swirl to coat. Add onion and celery; cook 5 minutes, stirring occasionally. Remove from heat. Combine shrimp and crab in a large bowl. Stir in onion mixture, remaining black pepper, remaining parsley, cheese, and egg whites.

(continued)

Add the egg and stir gently. Add panko and stir gently again. Form the cakes into ½" thick patties. Heat skillet over medium high heat and remaining oil to the pan. Add patties and cook 3 minutes or until lightly browned, gently turn over, cook another 3 minutes or until done. Serve with the sauce. Makes 8 cakes, 2 cakes per serving.

Notes: Per serving: Calories 438, Protein 26 g, Carbohydrates 44 g, Fat 17 g, Sodium 520 mg, Potassium 418 mg, Phosphorus 316 mg.

Crabmeat Imperial

Vegetable cooking spray

½ c celery, chopped

½ c green pepper, chopped

½ c red pepper, chopped

1 tsp prepared mustard

ground white and red pepper to taste

2 T fresh parsley

⅛ tsp hot sauce

2 eggs, beaten

⅓ c low fat mayonnaise

½ c crab meat

½ c sea legs or surami (imitation crab meat)

Coat a large skillet with cooking spray and heat over medium high heat. Add celery, green and red peppers, and sauté until tender. Remove from the heat and stir in parsley, mustard, white and black pepper, and hot sauce. Set aside. Combine eggs and mayonnaise in a small bowl until smooth, and set aside. Add vegetable mixture to the mayonnaise mixture and stir well. Add the crabmeat and sea legs and stir gently. Spoon the crabmeat mixture into 8 baking shells. Arrange shells on a baking sheet and bake at 375ºF for 20-25 minutes. Serves 8.

Notes: Per serving: Calories 144, Carbohydrates 12 g, Protein 12 g, Fat 5 g, Sodium 326 mg, Potassium 282 mg, Phosphorus 148 mg.

Linguine With Clam Sauce

There is nothing like the smell of olive oil and garlic cooking to get everyone ready for dinner. This recipe can be "jazzed" up with the addition of a couple shrimp, scallops, crab, or even lobster.

12	oz linguine pasta uncooked
3	T olive oil
3	T fresh parsley, chopped
4	garlic cloves, chopped
6½	oz can chopped clams
1	T lemon juice
½	tsp oregano
¼	tsp crushed red pepper flakes
1	tsp black pepper
3	oz shredded Parmesan cheese, divided

Cook linguine according to package directions. Drain and cover to keep warm. In a large skillet, heat olive oil over medium heat. Add garlic, stirring for 30 seconds. Add clams, parsley, lemon juice, oregano, crushed red pepper, black pepper, and half of the Parmesan cheese. Reduce heat to low and simmer for 5 minutes. Put linguine on plates and top with clam sauce. Top the pasta with the remaining Parmesan cheese and garnish with fresh parsley. Serves 4.

Notes: Per serving: Calories 500, Carbohydrates 66 g, Protein 19 g, Fat 17 g, Sodium 459 mg, Phosphorus 337 mg, Potassium 239 mg.

Greek-Style Shrimp Scampi

I tested this recipe for a large group of friends and it received a standing ovation. The feta cheese melts over the scampi sauce and the lemon juice makes the flavors come alive.

4	tsp olive oil
7	cloves garlic, crushed
¼	c fresh parsley
8	oz can whole, garlic-flavored tomatoes, drained and coarsely chopped
1	lb shrimp, uncooked, tail and shell off
3	oz feta cheese, crumbled
2	T lemon juice
12	oz spaghetti noodles, dry

Preheat oven to 400ºF. Cook pasta according to package instructions. Heat oil in a large skillet over medium heat. Add garlic and sauté for 30 seconds. Add half the parsley and all of the tomatoes. Reduce heat and simmer for 10 minutes. Add shrimp, and cook 5 minutes. Pour mixture into a 13x9 inch-baking dish. Sprinkle with feta. Bake at 400ºF for 10 minutes. Sprinkle with the remaining parsley, 2 T lemon juice, and black pepper. Serve over pasta. Serves 6, 1 c pasta and ½ c sauce.

Notes: Per serving: Calories 375, Carbohydrates 48 g, Fat 8 g, Protein 26 g, Sodium 378 mg, Phosphorus 308 mg, Potassium 426 mg.

Quick And Elegant Sole With Shrimp

This recipe takes less than 10 minutes to prepare, but the flavor is that of a special event meal. Serve with rice and a fresh salad tossed with olive oil vinaigrette.

1	lb filet of Sole, Flounder, Orange Roughy or Tilapia
¼	c raw shrimp, tail and shell off and cut into large pieces
3	T plain breadcrumbs
¼	tsp black pepper
2	T lemon juice
1	c mushrooms, sliced
2	T mayonnaise
¼	c green onions, sliced into small pieces
2	cloves garlic, minced
1	T butter, slightly melted
¼	c white wine

Place half of the fish in an even layer in a casserole dish. Sprinkle the fish evenly with half of the shrimp, breadcrumbs, pepper, lemon juice, and sliced mushrooms. Repeat the layers. Combine mayonnaise, green onions, garlic, and softened butter. Dot the mayonnaise mixture over the mushrooms and drizzle with the white wine.

Bake covered at 350ºF for 30 minutes or until the fish flakes easily. Uncover the last 5 minutes while the mayonnaise mixture puffs up and browns a bit. Serves 5.

Notes: Per serving: Calories 190, Carbohydrates 8 g, Fat 6 g, Protein 24 g, Sodium 202 mg, Phosphorus 253 mg, Potassium 495 mg.

Border-Style Shrimp

1½   c white onion, chopped

cooking spray

1   tsp ground cumin

1   tsp chili powder

1½   lb shrimp, peeled

3   cloves garlic, minced

1   T olive oil

1   T butter

⅛   tsp hot sauce

¼   c lime juice

lime wedge as a garnish

¼   c green onions

Heat a large nonstick skillet coated with vegetable cooking spray over medium heat and 1 T olive oil. Add onions and sauté 3 minutes. Add cumin, chili powder, shrimp, and garlic, and sauté for 4 minutes. Remove from the heat and add butter and hot sauce and stir until the butter melts. Stir in lime juice and green onions, garnish with lime wedges and serve. Makes 4 servings, about 1 c each. Serve over rice.

Notes: Per serving: Calories 111, Carbohydrates 6 g, Protein 7 g, Fat 7 g, Sodium 72 mg, Potassium 160 mg, Phosphorus 82 mg.

Risotto With Vidalia Onion and Shrimp

8   oz shrimp, remove shell and tail

3   tsp olive oil

2   c Vidalia onions, chopped

1½   c uncooked Arborizo rice

28   oz vegetable broth (page 44)

5   cloves garlic, minced

2   oz feta cheese, crumbled

¼   c fresh parsley

Heat oil in a saucepan over medium heat. Add onion and garlic and sauté for 1 minute. Stir in rice. Add ½ of the heated broth, and cook until the liquid is nearly absorbed, stirring often. Add remaining broth, ½ c at a time stirring constantly until each portion of broth is nearly absorbed before adding the next. After 10 minutes, drop the shrimp into the rice and allow them to cook while more broth is being added. Add broth ½ cup at a time until you have used all of the broth. This process will take about 20 minutes total. After 20 minutes, when the rice has absorbed all the broth, remove the saucepan from the heat. Stir in 1 oz of the feta and all of the parsley. Spoon the risotto into a serving bowl and sprinkle with the remaining feta and black pepper to taste. Makes 5 servings, 1 cup each.

Once you learn to make risotto you can alter the ingredients. For example, you can substitute a little white wine for broth or add different vegetables or protein.

Notes: Per serving: Calories 450, Carbohydrates 72 g, Protein 19 g, Fat 9 g, Sodium 320 mg, Phosphorus 265 mg, Potassium 470 mg.

Scallops With Zucchini And Mushrooms

4	T olive oil
4	small zucchini, cut into thin strips
6	fresh mushrooms, thinly sliced
3	cloves garlic, minced
¼	tsp black pepper
1	lb scallops
2	T lemon juice
2	T fresh parsley

In a large frying pan, heat the oil over medium heat, swirling to coat the pan. When the oil is hot add the zucchini and mushrooms. Stir and toss until they are tender-crisp, about 2-3 minutes. Add the garlic and sit for 1 minute. Transfer to a bowl and set aside. Add more oil to the pan and heat, add half the scallops and toss until just tender, 2-3 minutes. Transfer to the bowl with the vegetables. Add the remaining oil to the pan and heat. Add the rest of the scallops. Return all the scallops and vegetables to the pan. Heat for about 30 seconds, add black pepper and lemon juice, stir. Transfer to a serving dish and sprinkle with parsley and garnish with lemon slices. Serves 4.

Notes: Per serving: Calories 229, Carbohydrates 7 g, Protein 20 g, Fat 13g, Sodium 184 mg, Phosphorus 269 mg, Potassium 442 mg.

Singapore Noodles
With Shrimp

5	oz rice noodles
¼	tsp cumin seeds
⅛	tsp coriander seeds
⅛	tsp mustard seeds
1	garlic clove
⅛	tsp ground red pepper
1	c green onions, cut into 1" pieces
3	T vegetable oil
2	slices turkey bacon, chopped into small pieces
	cooking spray
1	lb raw shrimp, peeled and deveined
2	T low sodium soy sauce
1	T rice wine vinegar
2	tsp chili garlic sauce
1	T Hoisin sauce
1½	tsp grated fresh ginger, divided
½	c julienne cut red bell pepper

Preheat broiler. Soak noodles in hot water for 2 minutes. Drain well. Combine cumin, coriander, mustard seeds, and garlic clove in a spice grinder or coffee grinder. Pulse until ground, and stir in red pepper. Combine green onions, 2 tsp oil, and bacon in a small bowl. Place onion mixture on a rimmed baking

(continued)

sheet coated with cooking spray. Broil 5 minutes. Add shrimp to mixture and toss. Arrange shrimp in a single layer and broil 5 minutes until shrimp and bacon are done. Transfer this mixture to a bowl using a slotted spoon. Add black pepper. Combine cumin mixture, soy sauce, vinegar, Hoisin sauce, chili garlic sauce, and ½ tsp ginger. Heat the remaining 1 T of oil, and then add bell pepper and the remaining ginger. Sauté 45 seconds and add to shrimp mixture. Return skillet to medium high heat, add soy sauce mixture and noodles, cook 1 minute or until thoroughly heated, tossing to coat. Place ¾ c noodles on each of 4 plates and top with ¼ of the shrimp. Serve immediately. Serves 4.

This is not as low sodium as I usually strive for, but it is greatly improved over a restaurant meal you might indulge in instead.

Notes: Per serving: Calories 242, Carbohydrates 35 g, Protein 13 g, Fat 5 g, Sodium 543 mg, Potassium 220 mg, Phosphorus 182 mg.

Acorn Squash Stuffed With Rice Pilaf

⅔   c brown rice

⅓   c water

     cooking spray

1   acorn squash, cut in half and seeded

1   T olive oil

½   onion, minced

1   apple, unpeeled and chopped

¼   c dried cranberries

     pepper to taste

Combine rice and water in a medium saucepan and bring to a boil. Reduce heat to low, cover and cook for 40 minutes. Meanwhile, preheat the oven to 400ºF. Line a baking sheet with foil and spray with cooking spray. Place the squash on the sheet cut side down. Roast the squash for 35 to 40 minutes, or until you can easily insert a fork into them from the skin side. While the squash is cooking, heat olive oil in a skillet, add onion and stir until cooked, about 5 minutes. Add chopped apples and cranberries. Cover and cook for 12 minutes until the apple is soft. Mix the onion, apple, and rice together. Halve the squash halves (giving you 4 pieces). To serve: Put 1 piece of squash on a plate and place ¼ of the rice mixture on top of it.

If you are not following a potassium restriction diet, then you may have an entire half of a squash. However, if you need to keep your potassium down, then you should stick with ¼ of a squash. Serves 4. This recipe is also delicious made with white rice and lots of curry spice.

Notes: Per serving: Calories 188, Carbohydrates 42 g, Protein 4 g, Fat 1 g, Sodium 5 mg, Potassium 461 mg, Phosphorus 155 mg.

Rice Primavera

2½ c homemade chicken broth (page 45) or low sodium store broth

1   c white rice

2   T olive oil

3   cloves garlic, minced

2   T shallots, minced

1   c green beans, but into 3" pieces

1   c carrots, diced

1   c frozen green peas, thawed

1   c zucchini or yellow squash, diced

¼   c fresh Parmigiano-Reggiano cheese and a bit more to serve on the side

1   T green scallion tops

1   T fresh parsley

Once the broth is boiling stir in the rice. Cook covered over low to medium heat until the rice is tender and broth is absorbed, about 25 minutes. Meanwhile, heat oil in a large skillet. Add the garlic and cook 1 minute. Add shallots, green beans, and diced carrots. Sauté the vegetables for 2 minutes stirring frequently. Stir in the peas; cover and cook for another 2 minutes. Remove from the heat and stir in the zucchini. Cover and let stand off the heat. Stir the cheese into the cooked rice until creamy, and then add rice to the skillet and stir until blended with vegetables. Add black pepper to taste. Place into a serving dish, top with scallion tops and parsley. Serve with Parmesan cheese on the side. Makes 4 servings.

Notes: Per serving: Calories 383, Carbohydrates 55 g, Protein 14 g, Fat 10 g, Sodium 275 mg, Potassium 295 mg, Phosphorus 208 mg.

Zucchini and Cheese Casserole

3   lbs zucchini, unpeeled and cut into 1" chunks

1   c low fat cottage cheese

4   oz shredded Monterey Jack cheese

2   eggs or 2 egg whites, beaten

1   tsp dill seeds

½   c dried breadcrumbs

1   T butter, cut up

Preheat the oven to 350ºF. In a saucepan, simmer the zucchini chunks in very lightly salted water for 5 minutes. Drain well. In a large casserole dish combine the zucchini with the cottage cheese, Monterey Jack cheese, eggs, and dill seeds. Bake the casserole uncovered at 350ºF for 15 minutes. Sprinkle the breadcrumbs on top of the zucchini mixture, dot with butter and bake another 15 minutes uncovered so it is able to brown on top. Serves 6.

Notes: Per serving: Calories 166, Carbohydrates 13 g, Protein 12 g, Fat 7 g, Sodium 389 mg, Potassium 301 mg, Phosphorus 165 mg.

Citrus Barbecue Tofu

2	14 oz packages of extra firm tofu cut into 8 or 9 slices
4	T lemon juice
½	c Sunny Delight orange flavor*
4	T maple syrup
4	T apple cider vinegar
2	T olive oil
3	garlic cloves, minced
2	tsp rosemary
3	tsp low sodium soy sauce
	black pepper to taste

Whisk all ingredients except the tofu in a bowl to make the marinade. Put the tofu slices in a flat dish and pour the marinade over it. Cover and refrigerate for 4 hours, allowing the flavors to penetrate the tofu. Turn the grill on medium and brush lightly with olive oil. Grill the tofu slices and baste with the extra marinade. Cook 5 minutes on each side. Serves 4.

*Sunny Delight is a low potassium orange juice substitute.

Notes: Per serving: Calories 208, Carbohydrates 16 g, Protein 11 g, Fat 10 g, Sodium 162 mg, Potassium 182 mg, Phosphorus 168 mg.

Orange Glazed Tofu
With Sesame Rice

2	12 oz packages of water-packed extra firm light tofu
¼	c Sunny Delight orange flavor*
2	T low sodium soy sauce, divided
1	T rice vinegar
2	tsp honey
1	tsp chili sauce with garlic
½	tsp fresh ginger, grated
	cooking spray
1	c frozen green peas, thawed
2	tsp sesame oil
1	c carrots, grated
½	c green onions, thinly sliced
2	c hot cooked long grain white or brown rice
2	T sesame seeds, toasted

Cut tofu into ¾" chunks. Arrange tofu pieces in a single layer on several layers of paper towels, cover with more paper towels. Place a cutting board on top of the paper towels and let stand 15 minutes. Combine Sunny Delight, 1 T soy sauce, rice vinegar, honey, ½ tsp chili garlic sauce, and ginger in a shallow bowl stirring with a whisk. Remove cutting board and paper towels from tofu and add the tofu slices to the

marinade turning in the dish to coat well. Cover and marinate at room temperature for 30 minutes, turning over after 15 minutes. Heat a grill pan over medium heat. Coat the pan with cooking spray. Drain tofu and discard the marinade. Add tofu to the pan and cook 3 minutes until lightly brown. Turn the tofu over and cook another 2 minutes. Set aside and keep warm. Heat oil in a medium nonstick skillet over medium heat. Add peas, carrots, and onions cooking 2 minutes. Stir in the remaining soy sauce, and the remaining chili garlic sauce. Add cooked rice, cook 2 minutes or until heated. Stir in sesame seeds. Place 1 c rice mixture on each plate and arrange 3 tofu slices on top of the rice. Serves 4.

*Sunny Delight is a low potassium orange juice substitute.

Notes: Per serving: Calories 314, Carbohydrates 39 g, Protein 13 g, Fat 13 g, Sodium 320 mg, Potassium 324 mg, Phosphorus 224 mg.

Angel Hair Pasta Primavera

This is a decadent dish for those who wish to gain weight or who worry about weight loss.

5	oz slender asparagus stalks, bottoms removed and sliced into 1" pieces
5	oz summer squash, sliced
½	c broccoli florets
3	T olive oil
4	oz mushrooms, sliced
4	oz turkey bacon, cut into small pieces
3	oz spring onions, green and white parts sliced
3	garlic cloves, minced
1	c heavy whipping cream
⅓	c white wine
¼	tsp nutmeg
¼	tsp black pepper
12	oz angel hair pasta, dry
½	c Parmesan cheese, shredded

In a 3 to 4 quart pan, cook asparagus, squash, and broccoli in 1 quart boiling water, uncovered, for 2 minutes. Drain vegetables and set aside. Heat olive oil in a wide frying pan over medium heat, add mushrooms and cook until they begin to brown, 3-5 minutes. Add turkey bacon, onions, and garlic.

Continue cooking until the onions are soft and bright green. Add cream, wine, nutmeg, and pepper. Increase heat to high and bring to a low boil, stirring often. Meanwhile, in a 5-6 quart saucepan cook pasta in boiling water until just tender to the bite. Drain well. To cream mixture, add vegetables and the cheese, stir gently. Remove from heat, add pasta, and mix gently until pasta is coated with the sauce. Serves 6.

Notes: Per serving: Calories 422, Carbohydrates 50 g, Protein 14 g, Fat 18 g, Sodium 409 mg, Phosphorus 220 mg, Potassium 424 mg.

If you are a diabetic and looking for a "less glycemic" pasta try Dreamfields Pasta. It is 65% less glycemic that regular pasta and it has a delicious taste.

Pasta with Caramelized Squash and Fresh Herbs

This is a perfect autumn dish. Even my daughter, who was not too eager to try the squash, loved the recipe. Fresh herbs really bring out the flavor, which is especially important when not using salt in recipes.

4	T butter
1	c raw butternut squash, diced into 1" pieces
2	T sugar
4	oz chicken broth (page 45)
3	T shallots, finely diced
⅛	tsp ground nutmeg
⅛	T fresh ground sage
1	tsp lemon juice
2	T fresh parsley
1	oz fresh Parmesan cheese, shredded
8	oz bow tie pasta, uncooked

Melt 3 T butter in a large skillet over medium heat. Add the squash in a single layer and cook without stirring for 6 minutes. Flip squash and cook other side for 4 minutes. Add sugar, broth, and pepper. Cover and cook 2-3 minutes. Transfer to a bowl. In the same skillet melt 1 T butter.

Cook shallots, nutmeg, and sage for 1 minute. Turn off the heat and add lemon juice, parsley, and squash. Add black pepper to taste. Meanwhile, cook bow tie pasta according to package directions. Drain well and put in a bowl. Top pasta with squash and sauce, and sprinkle with Parmesan cheese. Serves 4.

Notes: Per serving: Calories 389, Carbohydrates 55 g, Protein 12 g, Fat 15 g, Sodium 106 mg, Phosphorus 174 mg, Potassium 306 mg.

Mock Sausage Noodle Tomato Casserole

1   8 oz package of broad egg noodles or yolk free egg noodles

2   T olive oil

1   onion, chopped

2   cloves garlic, minced

1   package of "Gimme Lean Sausage", usually found frozen

2   tsp ground oregano

2   tsp ground basil

½   c low fat cottage cheese

2   T Asiago cheese

2   T freshly grated Parmesan cheese

3   oz canned tomato sauce

Add noodles to boiling water. I recommend using bow tie, rigatoni, or twist pasta and not fragile pasta such as angel hair. Cook the noodles until they are just al dente. Drain the pasta and heat the olive oil in a large skillet. Add the onion and garlic. Add the "Gimme Lean Sausage" crumbles, oregano, basil, cottage cheese and tomato sauce. Cover the pan and let simmer a few minutes. Add the noodles and heat thoroughly. Just before serving, top with the Asiago cheese. Asiago cheese melts beautifully and adds richness to the flavor. The "Gimme Lean Sausage" is a great ground beef or ground turkey substitute, and a subtle way to add soy to your diet.

(continued)

I do take liberties by using some foods that you may have read are not in your diet. In this case, I added 3 oz of tomato sauce. Because this recipe serves 4 people each person gets less than 1 oz of tomato sauce. Most of the potassium in this recipe comes from the soy. All protein sources are a considerable source of potassium, but protein is necessary for our diet, so it has been calculated in for you. Serves 4.

Notes: Per serving: Calories 383, Carbohydrates 37 g, Protein 26 g, Fat 15 g, Sodium 373 mg, Potassium 375 mg, Phosphorus 407 mg.

Vegetable Fried Rice

A colorful and delicious one-pot meal.

3	c cooked white rice
2	eggs
4	T olive oil
1	c broccoli florets
½	c carrots, chopped
½	c mushrooms, sliced
1	c sweet white or yellow corn, fresh or frozen
1	tsp sherry
¼	c Asian chicken broth (page 45)
2	T light soy sauce
¼	c spring onions, chopped

Heat 1 T olive oil in a wok or large skillet. Meanwhile, beat the eggs in a bowl. Add the eggs to the skillet stirring continuously until soft curds form, about 1 minute. Transfer to a bowl and set aside. Add another 1 T oil to the pan over high heat, and add broccoli, carrot, and mushrooms. Stir and toss every 15-20 seconds until the vegetables begin to soften, 2-3 minutes. Add the sherry and cook for 1 minute. Add the corn and stir, cooking for 1 minute. Remove the vegetables and put them in the bowl with the eggs. Add the remaining oil. When it is hot add the cooked rice and stir every 30 seconds for 5 minutes or until lightly browned. Add the soup stock, soy sauce, and green onions, and stir to combine. Add the reserved vegetables and egg. Stir until the rice mixture is heated through about 1 minute longer. Serves 4.

Notes: Per serving: Calories 431, Carbohydrates 65 g, Fat 16 g, Protein 8 g, Sodium 184 mg, Phosphorus 305 mg, Potassium 434 mg.

Chiles Rellenos Casserole

½	lb ground turkey
1	c onion, chopped
2	tsp ground oregano
2	tsp ground cumin
3	garlic cloves, minced
¼	tsp black pepper
8	oz refried beans, canned
8	oz whole green chilies, drained and cut lengthwise into quarters
4	oz Monterey Jack cheese
1	c corn, fresh or frozen
⅓	c flour
1⅓	c skim milk
2	eggs, lightly beaten
2	egg whites, lightly beaten
	hot sauce to taste

Preheat oven to 300ºF. Cook ground turkey and onion in a nonstick skillet over medium heat until browned, stirring to crumble the ground turkey. Remove the pan from heat; add oregano, cumin, garlic, black pepper, and refried beans. Stir well and set aside. Arrange half of the green chilies in an 11x7 inch-baking dish. Top with half the cheese. Spoon mounds of the turkey mixture over the cheese gently, leaving a ¼ inch border around the edge of the dish. Top with corn. Arrange remaining green chilies over corn and top with the remainder of the cheese. Put flour in a bowl, and gradually add milk, hot sauce, eggs, and egg whites. Stir with a whisk until blended. Pour over casserole. Bake at 350ºF for 1 hour and 5 minutes, or until set. Let stand 5 minutes, garnish with green onions and fresh cilantro. Serves 6.

Notes: Per serving: Calories 334, Carbohydrates 39 g, Fat 12 g, Protein 19 g, Sodium 309 mg, Phosphorus 327 mg, Potassium 462 mg.

Pasta With Fresh Tomato Sauce

3	small tomatoes or 2 large tomatoes
4	large garlic cloves, peeled but left whole
1	small hot red or green chili, chopped or red pepper flakes (¼ tsp)
½	c FRESH basil, coarsely chopped
½	c olive oil
1	lb penne or other tubular pasta
2	oz Fontina cheese
½	c freshly grated Parmesan cheese

Wash and wipe the tomatoes. Remove cores and chop tomatoes. Put garlic, chopped chili, basil, pepper, and olive oil in the bowl with the tomatoes. Let stand at room temperature for several hours, or chill overnight. Return to room temperature before serving. Cook pasta according to the package directions. Grate the Fontina cheese using a coarse blade. Drain the pasta when it is done cooking. Spoon off about ¼ c of the oil from the tomato sauce bowl and add it to the pasta. Add the Parmesan cheese and toss. Add half the remaining sauce and Fontina cheese and toss. Serve in soup bowls with the remaining sauce on top.

Serves 4.

From working with CKD patients over the years I know how much they miss the traditional tomato sauce. An authentic Italian tomato sauce can use as many as a dozen tomatoes, making it usually too high in potassium to be part of their diet. I looked for a long time to give my patients an acceptable substitute and I hope you like this as much as I do.

Notes: Per serving: Calories 434, Carbohydrates 22 g, Protein 10 g, Fat 35 g, Sodium 187 mg, Potassium 190 mg, Phosphorus 135 mg.

Breakfast

Spanish French Toast

2	c low fat or skim milk
2	eggs
3	T sugar
2	tsp ground cinnamon
2	tsp vanilla
2	T confectioners sugar
4	slices hearty peasant bread
2	T olive oil

In a bowl large enough to soak the bread, whisk together the milk, eggs, granulated sugar, 1 tsp of the cinnamon, and vanilla. Combine the remaining teaspoon of cinnamon with the confectioners sugar in a small bowl and set aside. Dip the bread in the batter to soak it well and allow it to soak until all the liquid has been absorbed, about 15 minutes. Heat the oil in a nonstick skillet over medium high heat. Lightly brown the bread, cooking in batches, use more oil if needed. Place 2 pieces of French toast on each plate and sprinkle with the cinnamon sugar mixture. Serve immediately. Serves 4.

I have provided you with a few French toast recipes, because pancakes and waffles use a lot of baking powder to plump them up. Baking powder has an additive, which is high in a type of phosphorous that is particularly inflammatory to the kidneys. French toast is a much healthier breakfast option.

Notes: Per serving: Calories 233, Protein 9 g, Carbohydrates 26 g, Protein 9 g, Fat 10 g, Sodium 260 mg, Potassium 260 mg, Phosphorus 206 mg.

French Toast with Fruit

French Toast

1	loaf French bread
4	oz low fat cream cheese
½	c raspberry preserves or a flavor of your choice
1	c egg beaters or other egg substitute
1	c skim milk
1	T sugar or granulated Splenda or Stevia if Diabetic

Sauce

10	frozen raspberries or other frozen berry of your choice
¼	c sugar or granulated Splenda or Stevia if Diabetic
2	tsp cornstarch
	cooking spray

Spray bottom and sides of a 13x9 inch glass baking dish with cooking spray. Cut bread into 24 ¾ inch slices. Soften the cream cheese either by leaving it at room temperature for 1 hour or taking it out of its metallic wrapper and microwaving it for 10 seconds. Spread 12 slices of bread with the cream cheese. Spread the other 12 slices with the fruit preserves. Place the bread with fruit preserves over the bread with cream cheese to make 12 sandwiches. Arrange these sandwiches in the baking dish. Press them together to make them fit. In a medium bowl, beat the egg product, milk, and 1 T sugar until well blended. Pour the mixture over the bread. Let stand until all the liquid is absorbed, about 15 minutes. Heat oven to 400°F. Cover dish with foil and bake for 10 minutes. Uncover and bake 15 to 20 minutes longer until brown. Meanwhile, mix sauce ingredients in a 2-quart saucepan until blended. Heat to boiling over medium heat

(continued)

and stir frequently. Boil for 30 seconds or until just thickened. Press through strainer to remove raspberry seeds. Serve sauce over the French toast. Serves 12.

Again, I have provided you with a few French toast recipes, because pancakes and waffles use a lot of baking powder to plump them up. Baking powder has an additive, which is high in a type of phosphorus that is particularly inflammatory to the kidneys. French toast is a much healthier breakfast option.

Notes: 2 bread slices per serving: Calories 197, Protein 6 g, Carbohydrates 39 g, Fat 2 g, Sodium 231 mg, Potassium 159 mg, Phosphorus 110 mg.

Baked French Toast With Berries

18	oz loaf of bread or ½ lb of a 1 lb French bread loaf, cut into ¾ inch slices
4	eggs beaten or 1 c of egg substitute
2	c skim milk
¼	c granulated sugar or granulated Splenda or Stevia if Diabetic
1	T vanilla
⅓	c brown sugar or Splenda brown sugar if Diabetic
¼	c butter
1	c fresh or frozen blueberries
1	c fresh sliced strawberries

Lightly grease a 3-quart glass dish. Arrange bread slices in the baking dish. In a large bowl, stir eggs or egg substitute, milk, granulated sugar, and vanilla. Slowly pour over the bread. Cover and chill for 8 hours or overnight. Combine flour, brown sugar, and cinnamon. Using a pastry blender or 2 knives, cut into butter until clumps the size of peas form. Cover and chill as well.

Before baking, preheat oven to 350ºF. Sprinkle blueberries over the bread, and sprinkle the flour mixture over the berries. Bake uncovered for 30 minutes. Let stand for 5 minutes and top with fresh strawberries cut into squares. Makes 8 servings.

(continued)

Once again, I have provided you with a few French toast recipes, because pancakes and waffles use a lot of baking powder to plump them up. Baking powder has an additive, which is high in a type of phosphorus that is particularly inflammatory to the kidneys. French toast is a much healthier breakfast option.

Notes: Per serving: Calories 184, Carbohydrates 27 g, Protein 9 g, Fat 5 g, Sodium 281 g, Potassium 301 mg, Phosphorus 126 mg.

Italian-Style Cheese Omelet

2	slices turkey bacon
2	T part skim ricotta cheese
2	T fresh basil, chopped
3	eggs
1	T water
2	tsp olive oil
2	T Parmesan cheese, grated

Chop the bacon. Combine bacon, basil, and ricotta cheese in a small mixing bowl. Stir to combine and set aside. In a separate mixing bowl, combine eggs, water, and pepper. Beat until combined. In a 9-inch nonstick skillet, add 2 tsp olive oil and swirl to cover. Add egg mixture and cook over medium heat until bottom of omelet is set and lightly browned, about 1-2 minutes. Spoon bacon and cheese mixture onto half of the omelet. Using a spatula, loosen omelet around edges.

Fold omelet in half using a pancake turner and slide onto a plate. Sprinkle with Parmesan cheese and serve. Makes enough to serve 2.

If you were wondering how many eggs per week you should consume I would stick with the American Heart Association's recommendation of 3 egg yolks per week.

Some research is showing that egg, soybean, and dairy protein is less harmful to the kidneys than we thought, but for now lets stick with 3 eggs per week.

Notes: Per serving: 140 calories, Carbohydrates 3 g, Protein 6 g, Fat 5 g, Sodium 120 mg, Potassium 70 mg, Phosphorus 120 mg.

Scrambled Huevos Rancheros

2   tsp olive oil

2   flour tortillas, 6" each

3   eggs

1   T sour cream

4   drops hot sauce

¼   c red pepper, chopped

¼   c green onions, chopped

½   medium tomato

1   oz Monterey Jack cheese with jalapeno peppers

In a small mixing bowl, combine eggs, sour cream, hot sauce, and black pepper. Beat with a fork until combined. In a 9" skillet, heat oil, add bell pepper and scallions and cook for 1 minute. Pour egg mixture over the peppers in the skillet and cook stirring frequently just until eggs are set, about 2 minutes. Stir in tomato and cook 30 seconds. Place tortilla, wrapped in a paper towel in the microwave and cook for 40 seconds until soft and warm. Divide egg mixture into each tortilla, sprinkle with jalapeno jack cheese and wrap tortilla. Makes 2 tortillas, 1 per person.

If you were wondering how many eggs per week you should consume I would stick with the American Heart Association's recommendation of 3 egg yolks per week.

Some research is showing that egg, soybean, and dairy protein is less harmful to the kidneys than we thought, but for now lets stick with 3 eggs per week.

Notes: Per serving: Calories 302, Carbohydrates 20 g, Protein 18 g, Fat 12 g, Sodium 334 mg, Potassium 224 mg, Phosphorus 272 mg.

Cereal Comparison

General Mills Fiber 1

Apple Cinnamon Mini Wheat

Instant Plain Oatmeal

Quaker Farina Cinnamon flavor

Quaker Women Apple Spice instant oatmeal

Cream of Wheat

Quaker Puffer Rice

Post Honey Bunches of Oats

½ c Fiber 1 Cereal: 180 mg potassium, 150 mg phosphorus, 105 mg sodium

¾ c Apple Cinnamon Mini Wheat: 166 mg potassium, 154 mg phosphorus, 20 mg sodium

½ c Instant oatmeal plain: 300 mg potassium, 360 mg phosphorus, 3 mg sodium (high phosphorus and potassium content most likely due to food additives added to enhance its cooking)

½ Quaker Farina Cinnamon flavor: 52 mg potassium, 44 mg phosphorus, 3 mg sodium

1 packed Quaker Spice Women's Cereal in Apple Spice: 138 mg potassium, 139 mg phosphorus, 319 mg sodium

(continued)

½ c Cream of Wheat: 36 mg potassium, 33 mg phosphorus, 7 mg sodium

1 c Quaker Puffer Rice: 60 mg potassium, 80 mg phosphorus, 5 mg sodium

¾ c Post Honey Bunches of Oats Honey flavor: 56 mg potassium, 43 mg phosphorus, 180 mg sodium

I tried to select plain cereals that offer some different options. When you start adding nuts, seeds, and raisins the potassium content drastically increases.

Notes: Food manufacturers are not required to list the potassium and phosphorus contents of their products, so not all data is available.

Some large differences also occur when different food flavor additives are added to cereals. For example, notice the difference in potassium and phosphorus contents in plain oatmeal versus apple spiced oatmeal.

Homemade Granola

2	c old-fashioned oats
2	oz slivered almonds
¼	c packed light brown sugar
¼	c vegetable oil
¼	tsp honey
1	tsp vanilla
¼	c dried cranberries
1	c corn flakes
1	c Rice Krispies

Preheat oven to 300ºF. In a bowl, mix oats, corn flakes, Rice Krispies, almonds, brown sugar, and cinnamon. In a saucepan, warm the oil and honey. Whisk in vanilla. Carefully pour the honey mixture over the oat mixture. Stir with a wooden spoon and finish with your hands, encouraging small clumps to form. Spread the granola on a baking sheet (15x10 inches) trying to make a thin, even layer. If the layer is too thick it will not be crispy. Bake for a total of 30 minutes, checking and stirring every 10 minutes. Transfer granola pan to a rack to cool. Mix in dried cranberries. Seal granola in an airtight container or bag.

You can store it at room temperature for 1 week or frozen for 3 months. Makes 9 ½ c servings.

Notes: Per ½ c serving of plain granola: Calories 280, Carbohydrates 51 g, Protein 3 g, Fat 8 g, Sodium 148 mg, Potassium 201 mg, Phosphorus 218 mg.

(continued)

You have different options milk for using with this granola:

4 oz of cow milk has 191 mg potassium and 123 mg phosphorus

4 oz of soy milk has 143 mg potassium and 63 mg phosphorus

4 oz of rice milk has 33 mg potassium and 67 mg phosphorus

4 oz of plain, skim yogurt has 312 mg potassium and 192 mg phosphorus

4 oz container of full-fat, plain yogurt has 165 mg potassium and 108 mg phosphorus

Soy yogurt is also high in potassium

Refer to your lab values to determine if you need to cut back on potassium, phosphorus or perhaps both to determine with milk or alternative is best for you.

If you like your granola a bit sweeter and you are not diabetic you can add more honey until it is just right for you.

Desserts

Ice Cream Options

(making the best of what is offered)

Better options with potassium under 500 mg per ½ c serving

Vanilla ice cream: 131 mg potassium, 69 mg phosphorus

Chocolate ice cream: 164 mg potassium, 71 mg phosphorus

Strawberry ice cream: 124 mg potassium, 66 mg phosphorus

Orange Sherbet: 71 mg potassium, 30 mg phosphorus

Vanilla bar covered with caramel and nuts: 129 mg
potassium, 62 mg phosphorus

Because nutritional information labels do not have to contain potassium and phosphorus this is a fairly lean list due to lack of information. Generally, fruit ices and sherbets are safe options and they come in a variety of flavors.

Ice cream desserts exceeding 500 mg potassium

McDonalds McFlurry Oreo Flavor

McDonalds McFlurry Original Flavor

Cookie Comparison

5 animal crackers: 50 mg potassium, 65 mg phosphorus

1 graham cracker: 9 mg potassium, 7 mg phosphorus

1 small oatmeal cookie (no raisins): 60 mg potassium, 64 mg phosphorus

3 Oreo cookies: 73 mg potassium, 54 mg phosphorus

1 large chocolate chip cookie: 82 mg potassium, 54 mg phosphorus

Note: Animal crackers and graham crackers are lower in sugar than the other options, and are allowed in moderation in the Diabetic diet. Raisins are very high in potassium.

Strawberries Dipped In Chocolate

This is a simple and healthy dessert that always hits the spot. Nothing is as delicious as sweet strawberries and rich chocolate. I often make this recipe for company and it is seen as a great delicacy.

1 package Bakers Chocolate in dark or milk chocolate

plump red strawberries, do not remove green tops

Microwave chocolate in a microwave safe bowl (glass) on high for 2 minutes, stirring after 1 minute. Do not overcook! The chocolate will continue to melt even after it is out of the microwave, just keep stirring. Using a bamboo shish kebob skewer, pierce the strawberry and dip it in the chocolate, twirling it to make sure it is well covered with the chocolate. Place on wax paper to dry. Let stand until the chocolate is firm. Serving size is 3 strawberries.

Make sure you do not overcook the chocolate, because once it gets thick and hard you cannot salvage it. It is better to undercook the chocolate and keep adding on just a few more seconds in the microwave at a time than to overcook the chocolate and have to throw it out and start all over again.

Notes: Per serving: Calories 107, Carbohydrates 14 g, Protein 1 g, Fat 6 g, Sodium 15 mg, Potassium 134 mg, Phosphorus 48 mg.

Lemon Sorbet with Blackberries

4   oz lemon sorbet or Italian ice

½   c fresh blackberries

This dessert is very refreshing and perfect for a hot summer evening.

You can garnish this dessert with a mint leaf and can substitute blueberries for blackberries if you prefer.

Notes: Per serving: Calories 120, Carbohydrates 30 g, Fat 0 g, Protein 1 g, Sodium 5 mg, Phosphorus 24 mg, Potassium 229 mg.

Watermelon Raspberry Ice Pops

2   c watermelon, seeded and diced

1   c fresh raspberries

⅓   c Splenda or Stevia granular

1   T lemon juice

1   T corn syrup

Place all ingredients in a blender and blend until smooth. Pour ingredients through a sieve into a bowl, trying to get the liquid but leaving the pulp behind. Pour into Popsicle molds and freeze for at least 6 hours. Makes 8 popsicles.

Notes: Per one pop: Calories 27, Fat 0 g, Protein 0 g, Fat 0 g, Carbohydrates 7 mg, Phosphorus 5 mg, Potassium 70 mg.

Cinnamon Crusted Apples

The aroma of these apples cooking is incredible.

4	medium granny smith apples, peeled, cored, and cut in half lengthwise
¼	c brown sugar firmly packed
2	T flour
½	tsp ground cinnamon
½	tsp ground nutmeg
2	T butter
1	egg white, beaten
	vegetable cooking spray

Preheat oven to 375°F. Combine brown sugar, flour, cinnamon, and nutmeg in a bowl. Stir well to combine. Cut in cutter until resembles coarse meal. Brush apples with egg whites and dredge them in brown sugar mixture. Place apples cut side down on an 11x7 inch pan coated in cooking spray. Add water to pan enough so apples are sitting in ½ inch of water, bake uncovered for 35 minutes or until apples are tender. Serves 8

Notes: Per serving: Calories 85, Carbohydrates 16 g, Protein 1 g, Fat 2 g, Sodium 35 mg, Phosphorus 16 mg, Potassium 120 mg.

Makeover Cheesecake with Blackberry Sauce

This dessert is incredibly light and delicious.

½	c low fat ricotta cheese
4	oz fat free cream cheese
4	T Splenda
1	tsp vanilla extract
1	c fresh raspberries
1	c fresh blackberries
2	T water

In a blender, combine the ricotta cheese, cream cheese, 2 T of Splenda, vanilla, and raspberries. Process until smooth, and transfer to a bowl. Rinse out the blender, add blackberries, water, and the remaining 2 T Splenda. Pulse to chop the blackberries. Divide half of the raspberry-cheese mixture among four dessert goblets. Top each goblet with half of the blackberry sauce. Add the remaining raspberry mixture and top with the remaining sauce. Garnish with a few raspberries. Chill for at least an hour in the refrigerator. Serves 4.

Notes: Per serving: Calories 71, Carbohydrates 8 g, Fat 2 g, Protein 5 g, Sodium 129 mg, Phosphorus 127 mg, Potassium 136 mg.

Applesauce Carrot Cake

1½   c white flour

½   c whole wheat pastry flour

⅔   c sugar

2   tsp baking soda

1½   tsp cinnamon

½   tsp nutmeg

¾   c unsweetened applesauce

¼   c vegetable oil

3   large eggs

3   c carrots, grated

     cooking spray

Preheat oven to 350ºF. Combine white and wheat flour, sugar, baking soda, cinnamon, and nutmeg in a large mixing bowl. In another bowl, combine the applesauce, oil, and eggs and add them to the flour mixture. Stir until the ingredients are well blended. Add the carrots and mix again. Thoroughly coat a 9-inch tube pan with cooking spray. Pour the batter into the pan. Bake the cake for about 1 hour 10 minutes or until a toothpick inserted into the cake comes out clean. Set the cake pan on a wire rack for 5 minutes. Run a knife around the edges of the pan to loosen the cake and turn over on a serving platter. Serves 16.

I highly recommend that you bake for yourself when baked goods are called for. Commercially prepared cakes have too many food additives, which are harmful to the kidneys. Boxed mixes are slightly better, but homemade baking is the healthiest option due to the lack of food additives.

Notes: Per serving: Calories 225, Carbohydrates 24 g, Protein 3 g, Fat 13 g, Sodium 21 mg, Potassium 110 mg, Phosphorus 54 mg. This cake contains 5249 IU of Vitamin A, which is really impressive!

Pound Cake with Strawberries and Cream

This recipe is easy and delicious.

1	slice already prepared pound cake
½	c fresh strawberries
2	T frozen whipped topping (Cool Whip), thawed

Place pound cake on a dessert plate, and top with fresh strawberries and whipped topping.

Notes: Per serving: Calories 198, Carbohydrates 24 g, Protein 1 g, Fat 7 g, Sodium 123 mg, Phosphorus 65 mg, Potassium 110 mg.

Sock It To Me Cake

This truly is a "sock it to me" cake in terms of calories. I recommend it for those concerned with weight loss or who hope to gain weight. I do not recommend this recipe for Diabetics.

1	box yellow cake mix
1	c sour cream
⅓	c vegetable oil
2	tsp cinnamon
2	T brown sugar
1	c pecans, chopped
¼	c sugar
1	c powdered sugar
2	T milk
4	eggs
¼	c water

Preheat oven to 375°F. Remove 2 t of cake mix and set it aside in a small bowl. Mix with cinnamon, brown sugar, and pecans. In a large bowl, blend remaining cake mix, sour cream, oil, water, eggs, and sugar. Beat on high speed for 2 minutes. Pour 2/3 of the batter into a greased and floured Bundt pan. Sprinkle the cinnamon sugar mixture in the center of this as a middle layer and spread remaining batter on top. Bake for 45-55 minutes. Cool in pan for 25 minutes. Serving is 1/8 of cake.

Notes: Per serving: Calories 628, Carbohydrates 80 g, Fat 34 g, Protein 5 g, Sodium 450 mg, Phosphorus 275 mg, Potassium 178 mg.

Spicy Angel Cake
Topped with Pineapple

Fresh pineapple is wonderful all year long. Try the "gold" version – it is extra sweet.

1	box angel food cake mix
1	tsp ground cinnamon
½	tsp ground nutmeg
¼	tsp ground ginger
¼	tsp ground cloves
½	c fresh pineapple

Put angel food cake mix into a bowl and add spices. Prepare and bake according to package instructions. Invert, cool completely in the pan. Cut into 1" slices and serve with fresh pineapple. Serves 8, serving size is 1/8 of cake and ½ c fresh pineapple.

Notes: Per serving: Calories 250, Carbohydrates 34 g, Fat 0 g, Protein 2.4 g, Sodium 55 mg, Phosphorus 76 mg, Potassium 115 mg.

Quick, Sugar Free Jell-O Parfait

If you are Diabetic or want a lower calorie option then you should select sugar free Jell-O.

4	oz Sugar Free Jell-O any flavor
½	c fresh raspberries
2	T frozen whipped topping (Cool Whip), thawed

Prepare Jell-O according to package directions or buy ready made. Place raspberries on top and place Cool Whip on the raspberries. Makes 1 serving.

I read a review of this recipe in which someone complained that a book that hopes to be gourmet should not provide Jell-O recipes. Since I try to provide you with options and education this recipe is just my way of saying that when you want something sweet and easy Jell-O with raspberries and Cool Whip is a safe option. This should be especially useful for Diabetic patients who are more limited in their sweets choices.

Notes: Per serving: Calories 140, Protein 0 g, Carbohydrates 11 g, Fat 2 g, Sodium 10 mg, Phosphorus 20 mg, Potassium 113

INDEX OF RECIPES

How to Order

10 STEP DIET & LIFESTYLE PLAN

FOR HEALTHIER KIDNEYS

AVOID DIALYSIS

NIINA KOLBE RD CSR LD
BOARD CERTIFED SPECIALIST IN RENAL NUTRITION

I suggest both books to obtain the best results toward improving the health of your kidneys. Kidney Health Gourmet is meant to be a companion guide to The 10 Step Diet & Lifestyle Guide for Healthier Kidneys. In the 10 Step Guide you learn to interpret your own lab values you learn in depth about potassium, phosphorus and protein. This is necessary so you can better select the recipes from this book. Since CKD has 5 stages the dietary needs can vary a great deal.

For ordering information for The 10 Step Guide please visit www.kidneyhealthgourmet.com

Or send a check to Nina Kolbe for $20.00 ($ 15.00 for the book and $5.00 for shipping)

Nina Kolbe
215 E Street SE
Washington, DC 20003

Please send me one copy of The 10 Step Diet & Lifestyle Plan. I am enclosing a check for $20.00. Please ship to:

Get additional copies of this cookbook by returning an order form and your check or money order to:

Nina Kolbe
215 E Street SE
Washington, DC 20003
Email: ninakolbe@aol.com
www.kidneyhealthgourmet.com

❖ ❖ ❖ ❖ ❖ ❖ ❖ ❖

Please send _____ copies of:

Kidney Health Gourmet

$15.00 for the book and $5.00 for shipping. Enclosed is

my check or money order for $_____

Mail Books To:

Name

Address

City   State   Zip

❖ ❖ ❖ ❖ ❖ ❖ ❖ ❖

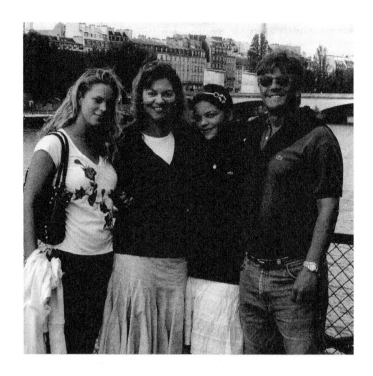

Nina Kolbe RD CSR LD has been a practicing dietician for over 22 years. She has chosen to specialize in kidney disease and became one of the first dieticians in the country to take the board certification exam to earn the title of Certified Renal Specialist. To maintain this certification 75 hours of continuing education must be maintained in the field of kidney disease. This assures patients that they are receiving the most up-to-date information from their health professional.

Nina maintains a private practice in the Washington DC Metro area. Many private physicians refer to her for nutritional counseling. In addition to a private practice, Nina also serves on the medical steering committee board of the National Institutes of Health (NIH) Kidney Disease Education Program, which is the medical steering committee of the National Kidney Foundation. She has been the chairperson for the Council of Renal Nutrition, a Renal Dietitian group, for 3 years.

Nina Kolbe has conducted research in the field of renal nutrition and presented this research at the National Kidney Foundation's Clinical Meetings. She has been published in the medical Journal *Nephrology News & Issues*. Nina Kolbe is frequently asked to give talks to health professionals in the field of renal nutrition.

Nina Kolbe's passion and dedication to her profession stems from her belief that early diagnosis and medical and nutritional intervention can delay the progression of kidney disease. Further, depending on when treatment is started, these lifestyle changes can help patients avoid dialysis.

CPSIA information can be obtained at www.ICGtesting.com
Printed in the USA
BVOW09s0839011115

424548BV00006B/66/P